DELIVERING HEALTH

POLICY T🌐 PRACTICE
Ethnographic Perspectives on Global Health Systems

SERIES EDITORS: Svea Closser, Emily Mendenhall, Judith Justice, & Peter J. Brown

Policy to Practice: Ethnographic Perspectives on Global Health Systems illustrates and provides critical perspectives on how global health policy becomes practice, and how critical scholarship can itself inform global public health policy. Policy to Practice provides a venue for relevant work from a variety of disciplines, including anthropology, sociology, history, political science, and critical public health.

Delivering Health

Midwifery and Development in Mexico

LYDIA Z. DIXON

VANDERBILT UNIVERSITY PRESS

Nashville, Tennessee

Library of Congress Cataloging-in-Publication Data

Names: Dixon, Lydia Zacher, 1980– author.
Title: Delivering health : midwifery and development in Mexico / Lydia
    Z. Dixon.
Description: Nashville : Vanderbilt University Press, [2020] | Series:
    Policy to practice | Includes bibliographical references and index.
Identifiers: LCCN 2020015428 (print) | LCCN 2020015429 (ebook) | ISBN
    9780826501134 (paperback) | ISBN 9780826501141 (hardcover) | ISBN
    9780826501158 (epub) | ISBN 9780826501165 (pdf)
Subjects: LCSH: Midwifery—Mexico. | Midwives—Training of—Mexico.
    | Midwifery—Study and teaching—Mexico.
Classification: LCC RG963.M6 D59 2020 (print) | LCC RG963.M6
    (ebook) | DDC 618.200972—dc23

LC record available at https://lccn.loc.gov/2020015428
LC ebook record available at https://lccn.loc.gov/2020015429

To my daughter Juno, and to all the midwives and the mothers

CONTENTS

ACKNOWLEDGMENTS

If the body of this book has not made it clear enough, I want to sincerely acknowledge the incredibly hard work done by the midwives, students, doctors, nurses, school administrators, public health workers, and activists whose struggles and achievements I have tried to make sense of here. Along the way, I met many people working in the world of women's health in Mexico with starkly divergent ideas about how to improve health outcomes and experiences; yet, despite their differences, they all reflected a passion for the women, families, and communities they were trying to help. The level of trust and openness extended to me was humbling, and I hope that I have done well by these diverse actors to represent their work.

While the research for this book took years, the final writing phases of it went relatively quickly. I want to thank the whole team at Vanderbilt University Press, but especially my editor, Zack Gresham, for his kindness, encouragement, and humor. His positivity kept me going during this process. I thank my reviewers, too, who made this book stronger through their careful readings and suggestions.

This book and the research that went into it could not have been completed without the following generous sources of funding: The Fletcher Jones Foundation Fellowship, Dr. Dard Magnus Rossell Memorial Award, UC Irvine Associate Dean's Fellowship, Inter-American Foundation Dissertation Research Fellowship, UC Irvine Center for Organizational Research, UC Irvine Global Health Framework Research and Travel Fellowship, UC MEXUS, and the UC Irvine Department of Anthropology. My initial introduction to professional midwifery in Mexico was funded through a University of Chicago Human Rights Internship Program. This book probably would not have been finished at all without the amazingly productive UC Irvine Steele/Burnand Anza-Borrego Desert Research Station writing retreat, where many feverish revisions were completed, and without the support of the Faculty Success Program (through the National Center for Faculty

Development and Diversity) provided by CSU Channel Islands. Large portions were also originally written over excellent coffee at the Catalina Island Brew House, my default office for many years.

This is a project that reflects my journey into the world of midwifery and women's health in Mexico as it has unfolded over the past eighteen years. As such, I must acknowledge the many mentors, teachers, colleagues, family members, and friends who supported my passion for this topic over the years, especially when it was not clear exactly where it would lead. While at UC Irvine, Michael Montoya, Leo Chavez, and Kris Peterson helped me frame this project and made it stronger. Hours of kitchen table and late-night phone conversations with the extremely knowledgeable and experienced women's health practitioners Alison Bastien, Annelle Taylor, and Kate Norman Frometa, who all work or have worked intimately with the populations described in this book, led to many breakthroughs in my analysis. I deeply value the feedback and support I have received along the way from colleagues and friends, including Caitlin Fouratt, Natali Valdez, Cheryl Deutsch Croshere, Taylor Nelms, Ather Zia, Sana Sadiq, Janny Li, Stevie Rea, Mark Durocher, Lee Ngo, Michael Hurley, Carole Browner, Vania Smith-Oka, Mounia El Kotni, and Veronica Miranda.

Finally, I thank my family for their patience, advice, and love throughout this process. My father, Christian Zacher, was a life-long scholar who passed away in 2019. His kind and thoughtful advice about writing and academia in general have helped me at every step of the way; his wife, Kay Bea Jones, and sister, Cathie Zacher, continue to extend that support. My mother, Judith Zacher, made me feel at home in hospital wards from a young age by taking me to work with her and showing me the creative and compassionate side of medicine; much of this book was also written at her kitchen table and was certainly inspired by her hard-earned perspective on health care. Mary Jo and Scott Dixon have been incredibly supportive of my family as I have tried to balance my work and motherhood. My siblings, Jessica Zacher Pandya and Sam Zacher, talked me through it all with humor and continue to inspire me with their own weighty achievements. Had I not picked up Jessica's dog-eared copy of Ina May Gaskin's *Spiritual Midwifery* while crashing on her couch one night back in the '90s, I may never have gone down this path. My brother-in-law, Mihir Pandya, was the first to even suggest I turn my interest in midwifery into a PhD in anthropology and has offered me much practical and thoughtful advice along the way. Meg Moir (not quite a sister, but close enough) was with me for this whole journey and kept me balanced when I got off course.

My daughter Juno was a part of this story from the beginning and tagged along with me during much of this research. My husband Pete and son Castor came along in the middle of it all, giving me the support to finish this project and inspiration to think about what comes next.

PROLOGUE

I studied birth for years before I experienced it myself. I thought I knew what to expect. Of course, experiencing birth was nothing like observing it, even as a doula helping others during labor.[1] When it came to the birth of my own child, I was completely surprised by the pain.

My hips were breaking apart. A searing, ripping pain took my breath away and seemed only slightly better when I yelled with my full lung capacity. When I looked at my midwife, Doña Guadalupe, she was gazing out into space, arms crossed, a slight smile on her face.[2] In other words, she was not nearly concerned enough to match my own level of panic. She could have been making a shopping list or thinking about what to cook for breakfast. As I lurched around the bedroom like a rabid animal, searching for some position to give me relief, she slowly pushed herself out of the chair where she had been waiting, watching, for the past hour. As she did so, she looked over at my doula and, with a slight chuckle, said to her in Spanish, "These gringas are always the screamers, right?"

I was pretty surprised by my own volume, but I felt like it would be literally impossible to be silent. I flashed back to the first birth I had seen, with this same midwife at the CASA (Center for the Adolescents of San Miguel de Allende) midwifery clinic where I was an intern right out of college a few years before. It was a small clinic in the central Mexican city of San Miguel de Allende, Guanajuato, and was associated with a professional midwifery school—the first of its type in the country. The birth I saw then was so serene and completely silent, but for a few measured grunts at the end. It had seemed achievable. I had certainly studied enough about birth (through doula trainings and volunteer work) in the intervening years to feel like I would get it right and do it gracefully. My own birth wouldn't even need to be in the CASA clinic, I had decided—which was why I was now laboring so loudly at home, across town from CASA. The thought passed as another contraction came on and I inhaled in anticipation of the unstoppable and out-of-control-feeling noises.

Doña Guadalupe made her way across the room and knelt down on the floor by the bed. She began to make a sort of floor nest of pillows and chucks pads. I watched her with one eye as I swayed and rocked, silently begging her to tell me it was time to deliver my first baby. She did not meet my eyes. Instead, she unhurriedly pulled items out of her small backpack: a cassette player, a candle, some brown glass homeopathic jars, a little kit of gloves and some other medical equipment, wrapped in sterile brown paper and sealed with masking tape. She lit the candle and set it on a table, then started the cassette player. At this point, she glanced up at me and explained, simply, "It is placenta noises, to soothe your baby when it comes."

Later, I would pause to wonder what the recording was and how it was made. But at that moment I thought, "That means that this is almost done!" And I nearly threw myself onto the floor in front of her. Sitting up was extremely painful, but given the preparations being made, I felt I could handle a few more minutes of hip-breaking pain if it was nearly over. However, as Doña Antonia quickly checked my cervix for the first time in hours, my hopes fell. She looked up at me with a serious expression and shook her head. "Your cervix is too swollen," she said. "You can't push the baby out like this, or it will tear."

The exhaustion of three days of labor and eight hours of intense pain crashed down on me with her proclamation. I began to cry, saying, "I can't do this!" For the first time, I saw my doula and Doña Guadalupe exchange worried glances, and I started to lose the little amount of control I had left. I bit down on a pillow, my muscles tense, unable to stay focused or breathe. That was when Doña Guadalupe said it was time to leave, to go to the CASA clinic. In my head I rebelled—I had planned this home birth and had been at it for days, I could not stop now!—but I did not have the strength to voice these thoughts. I let myself be led through the house and out to my doula's family jeep. I was loaded into the back, moaning and terrified of having to sit in a car for the twenty-minute drive across town to CASA. Doña Guadalupe sat up front, and I draped my body over her shoulders, grabbing onto her for dear life. It was five in the morning, and the streets of the sleepy town seemed eerily quiet, but anyone who saw us passing would have seen a strange sight: a packed jeep with a woman screaming obscenities into the neck of an older midwife, who was smirking as she commented mildly, "I don't speak English, but I do know what those words mean!"

We pulled up to the emergency entrance of the CASA clinic—a large, wooden door on a side street. I was helped out of the car and into the ward, which was empty except for a few midwifery students who were on duty that night. They looked at us, wide-eyed, as we made a loud entrance into the building. I recognized many of them from my time at CASA. I knew that they were all eager to be at more births: they jumped into action, readying a room and gathering supplies.

I was moving slowly, but even as I shuffled down the hall, I could feel that something in my body was different—later, Doña Guadalupe would laugh at the memory and say that the cobblestone streets had done the trick of getting my baby in position and pushing the cervix out of the way. "We should drive all our first-time moms around town on those streets," she joked, then suggested that "the hospital should get an old jeep just for the job."

I saw that Doña Guadalupe had hurried ahead of me and pulled on a set of scrubs. Her sudden transformation startled me, and I heard my doula ask her in a whisper (not quietly enough to avoid my ears) whether she was preparing for a possible cesarean. I had worked at CASA long enough to know that they had obstetricians on call who would come do the cesareans in their in-house operating room, but I had not expected to end up there myself. Doña Guadalupe replied that she had called the doctor and asked him to be ready just in case, but she was not making any decisions just yet. Still, her scrubs made me nervous.

I was led to birthing room number ten, where I lumbered up onto a bed. The room was so bright after the calm, candle-lit bedroom where I had been laboring. The lights were all on, and the wall was a glass door that was currently letting the full morning sunlight stream in. Suddenly there were students surrounding me, inserting an IV and asking me questions, pushing pillows behind my back and bringing carts into the room. I saw vials of medicines, aromatherapy bottles, and homeopathic remedies. Doña Guadalupe injected something into the IV. "What is that?" I managed to ask, between the contractions that were now coming nearly constantly. "It's for the pain," she told me, with a kind smile. At the time I thought, "Wonderful! Make the pain stop!" It didn't seem to do a thing, though. Later, she told me that it was only an over-the-counter pain medication, just to take off the edge.

A woman I had seen around CASA but had not yet met came into the room. She had a laptop under her arm and approached me to ask if she could observe my birth for a qualitative study on midwife births in Mexico. I remember feeling overwhelmed by the sudden onslaught of strangers in my space. But it didn't really matter anymore—I was so close to being done, one way or another. I told her sure, go ahead, and she set up her laptop in the corner of the room. Her fingers clicked out the details of the end of my labor as her eyes scanned the crowd. Later, I would learn that she was an anthropologist working for a Mexican public health organization, and I would find the parallels to my own future research remarkably coincidental.

Amid the chaos, I searched for my doula's eyes and locked onto them. She assured me that I was doing a good job. The midwife said she needed to check me one more time, and this time pronounced that I was fully dilated and ready to go. I began the serious business of pushing my baby out, continuing my loud yelling as I went. My daughter was born quickly then, a healthy and beautiful baby with big eyes that locked right onto mine as the midwife put her in my arms. "Well done!" said the midwife, kindly. I knew she was just being nice—I had been a noisy, panicked, cursing mess. But I had done well in the end, because this baby was perfect.

———————————

It has been thirteen years since that long night and hectic morning at CASA. In the intervening years I have spent a lot of time with Doña Guadalupe and a lot more time in those birthing rooms.[3] The rooms themselves have been painted and repainted, appointed with birthing stools and birthing ropes and—in one room—even a birthing tub. I've watched women labor in those rooms, and seen babies born, and have been the anthropologist in the corner and the woman holding the hand and saying, "You're doing a great job." Every time I am there, though, I pause at room ten and peek in, and I can feel the details of my own birth come rushing back to me (see Figure 1).

My birth did not mark the beginning of my interest in midwifery and women's health in Mexico. I had begun working with the CASA midwives four years prior, in 2002, through a post-college internship. Some days after my baby was born I thought back again to the first birth I had witnessed. It was just down the hall from room ten in CASA's birth center, at the start of that internship. The fact that the full memory did not surface during my own labor was a gift, because, while that first birth had been serene, it had nearly ended in a frightening way. I was called in to cool a laboring woman with a paper fan as she gave birth to her third child. She did so nearly silently, though with great exertion, as I fanned her face and murmured encouragement alongside a group of midwifery students, each of whom had a job to do. The baby came quickly, but I could tell immediately that all was not well: she was pale blue and silent. My knees weakened as my mind flashed to the worst possible outcome. But moments later the midwife was rubbing the

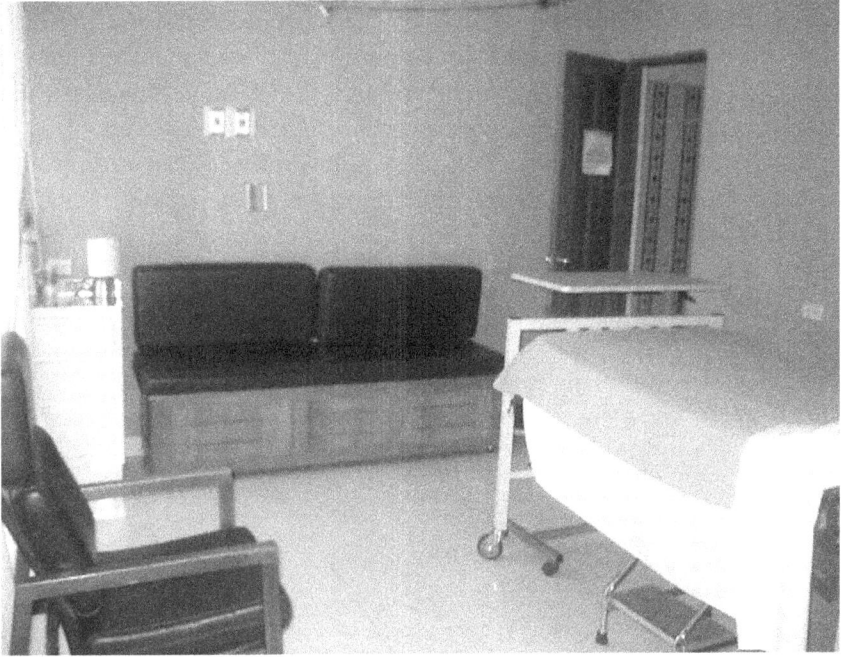

FIGURE 1: Room 10 at CASA's clinic. Photo by author.

baby, holding her upside down and saying, "*Vamos, bebé*" (Let's go, baby). The patient scrambled up onto her elbows to see what was wrong, and the students and I all held our breath as the midwife urged the baby on with her hands and her words. This process seemed to go on forever, but it was probably less than a minute until baby suddenly breathed in and cried out, turning pink and flailing her little arms. The mother cried out as well, in relief, and fell back as the midwife hurried the baby to the other room and a waiting supply of emergency oxygen.

I am not a midwife. I do not come from Mexico. Yet I have I lived most of my professional life in Mexico and the Western United States, working on a variety of reproductive health-related jobs, attending births as a doula, and learning about midwifery as much as possible. I went to graduate school soon after my daughter's birth at CASA, where I spent another four years shadowing midwives in bedrooms and clinics. But in writing this book about the persistence of midwifery in Mexico, I cannot help but think about my own role as a constant observer, much like the role of the midwife. I think back to my own experience that morning at the CASA midwifery clinic, with the midwife with one hand on the cell phone to call the obstetrician and the other hand on the homeopathic tablets. I think about the students eagerly learning from a traditionally trained professional. I am bemused by the anthropologist in the corner. I think about how the very threads traced through this book were there that bright morning in room ten: ideas of Western medicine and traditional knowledge, an educational model in progress, and the ever-present reality that things can go bad quickly, but that when things go well the results are beautiful.

This book is for my daughter, Juno, who came into the world on that significant morning. It is also dedicated to Doña Guadalupe, who is central to the chapters to follow. It is also for all those who were there in the room for my birth (you know who you are) and to those who are there for all the others.

Introduction

I never did find out exactly how the flat cardboard box full of vials of Pitocin had come to fill half a shelf in Juana's home; it certainly wasn't what I had expected to see after working my way through the chickens that walked in and out of her small adobe home in rural Oaxaca. I only knew that the presence of this drug—used to mimic the body's natural hormone, oxytocin, to force the uterus to contract, either during labor or in case of postpartum hemorrhage—reiterated for me the impossibility of neatly dividing "traditional" from "biomedical" knowledge, practice, or practitioners.

"What does this say?" the midwife asked me, holding one of the vials up to my face as she squinted at me through eyes that either could no longer read the tiny lettering on the bottle or perhaps could not read at all. "It's Pitocin," I assured her, although from what I could see the entire flat of vials contained the same thing. Before I had even finished clarifying this for her, she had found a new syringe packet in one of her many apron pockets, opened it, and was drawing the liquid into it. "I always inject my patients postpartum," she explained to me as she made her way to the bedside of a woman whose baby had been born there hours before. The woman was nursing her child and looked up, nonplussed, at Juana as she said, "We learned about it in a training; it prevents hemorrhage." Swiftly, Juana shifted the blankets, raised the woman's dress, and injected her in the thigh; she then repeated the whole process with her second patient in an adjoining bed. The patients hardly reacted to the procedure as they tended to their newborns.

Was *this* traditional midwifery—blindly injecting women with a powerful pharmaceutical as a matter of routine? This was a question that I ruminated on for the few days I spent with Juana, sleeping in the communal bedroom and helping with the patients when they needed food or water. We drank thick hot chocolate each morning, steamed large green squashes for a midday meal, and dipped crusty bread in coffee before bed. I accompanied Juana to the market, listened in as she chatted with the women of her town, trading news and giving out advice about pregnant relatives or friends. As we sat around her old wooden table in the evenings, I tried to ask the midwife about her work. Although she referred to herself as a *partera tradicional* (traditional midwife) she was vehement in her position against the kinds of "natural" remedies that I had heard linked to traditional midwifery in the region, such as teas, tinctures, or steam baths. Juana must have been near eighty years old, yet it was her much-younger neighbor, Elena, who later told me that *she* was the one in town who used plants and plant medicine. Women in their village know this, she told me: if you want traditional plant remedies, see the younger midwife; if you want drugs, see the elder.

To add to this juxtaposition, the two midwives' homes did not seem to align with their therapeutic approaches. Juana's simple two-room home was dark and cozy, filled nearly wall to wall with beds, piled high with thick blankets and holding laboring women or new mothers with their visiting older children and husbands. The bathroom was a wooden outhouse. Chickens wandered in and out of the open doors, and Juana's husband tended to their horse in the front garden. Elena's house, by contrast, was open, bright, and spacious. Elena invited me to visit after I had been at Juana's house for a few days. Compared to Juana's home, entering Elena's space felt like stepping forward in time—there was a television on, and children ran in and out of the sun-filled courtyard, playing with trucks. Yet Elena's plant remedies were hung in neat bundles in her herb room or packaged in small glass jars on a shelf. There were no signs of Pitocin, no syringe packets.

I accompanied Elena on a trip up the local mountains where she searched for a specific medicinal plant that was in season. She had me climb into the back of her family's pickup truck while she, her husband, and their small toddler rode in the cab. I held on tightly as we headed up windy mountain roads, stopping every mile or so to get out and search the hillsides by foot. We hiked around the scrub brush, and I felt my head spin as Elena pointed out and named each plant and described its various medicinal values. At one point, she ripped a stem off a plant and told me to chew on it. "It is a natural toothbrush that Indigenous people sometimes use to clean their teeth!" she explained, laughing at the face I made as I attempted a few tentative chews (it did not taste very good). Most plants she identified, she left where they were—she had enough of them, or it was not the right time to harvest them yet. That day, she was only collecting what she called *cardo santo* (holy thistle, or as it is called more commonly in English, blessed milk thistle). The plant was easy to spot (even for me, as inexperienced as I was), with its round and prickly flower, its pink petals spiking upwards. Elena explained that *cardo santo* has a variety of uses, from digestive remedies to helping increase milk production in breastfeeding women.

I came to know both Juana and Elena in 2003 when I was living in Oaxaca City, Oaxaca, in southern Mexico, and working on a cervical cancer prevention program—years before beginning my doctoral program in anthropology. I had moved to Oaxaca after first spending a year just out of college interning at a midwifery school and clinic called CASA (Centro Para los Adolescentes de San Miguel de Allende—Center for the Adolescents of San Miguel de Allende) located in the central Mexican city of San Miguel de Allende, Guanajuato. My time at CASA had piqued my interest in childbirth and midwives, and when I moved south to Oaxaca I helped start a grassroots midwifery study collective and began to meet and learn from local midwives. Shortly after I arrived, a local women's center helped organize an international midwifery conference. There, as I watched midwives from across the Americas come together and learn from each other, I understood for the first time both the diversity of midwifery practices and knowledge and the shared sense of struggle many midwives expressed facing.

They saw a real need for their services in their communities but described how they were up against a medical system that had been trying for decades to push them out. Nurses and public health workers were going door to door, telling their patients and patients' families that midwives—the women who had cared for generations of women in their communities—were dangerous and that the only safe way to birth was in state clinics or hospitals. They called midwives witches, said that they would kill the women's babies—or the women themselves. They promised safe births and good outcomes if the women would only come to the clinic instead.

Yet women were not always able to access these state facilities, and they were not always having good experiences and outcomes when they could. Midwives from across Mexico were increasingly coming together to share these stories and strategize about how to continue to help the women in their communities. The internet was certainly helping in their efforts to organize, and it was evident that their message had been heard widely by the range of midwives who were in attendance at the international midwifery conference in Oaxaca. It was during such gatherings that the idea for a national organization for advocacy and women's health-care reform began to circulate. Years later, while conducting the ethnographic fieldwork that informs the rest of this book, I would witness that organization come to fruition—the Mexican Midwifery Association (La Asociación Mexicana de Partería), but in those early days I watched as diverse midwives were just starting to build national networks and define their goals.

It was at that conference in Oaxaca that I met Juana and Elena, two very different midwives both living in the same small village about a half hour outside Oaxaca City. After speaking with them over lunch one day, I asked them if I could visit their village and see their consult rooms. I was surprised and grateful when they each said I could come and stay for a few days in their homes, observe them at work, and get to know their approaches to midwifery care.

In the years since, after spending many, many hours observing with and talking to midwives across Mexico, I continue to think about how those two midwives in one small town came to approach midwifery so differently: How one had access to Pitocin and syringes, and the other dried bundles of local herbs in her office. How they were each still sought out by women and families in their community, despite the concerted efforts of public health workers to redirect services to state clinics. How they each embraced the term "traditional midwife"—*partera tradicional*—but how it meant such very different things to each of them. As I came to know more midwives across Mexico in the years that followed, I continued to hear the term "traditional" contrasted with "professional" to distinguish midwifery practitioners, practices, ideologies, approaches to teaching and learning, and scopes of practice. Throughout my fieldwork, these were labels midwives used to differentiate themselves or each other, yet they were also used by politicians, physicians, the press, and the public to describe types of midwives. Often—importantly—the terms were used to mean different things by different people. On the surface, they reflected clear categories: traditional midwives used natural remedies and did not work in or with the hospital system, while professional midwives used some amount of biomedical interventions and may have been more officially tied to the system. Yet Juana called herself a traditional midwife, despite her reliance on biomedical tools and her distancing from natural remedies. Later, I would meet women who called themselves professional midwives who—in contrast to Juana—did not trust biomedical treatments and instead related professionalism to the use of a range of natural or alternative approaches.

Midwifery in Mexico is a diverse and dynamic profession that continues to persist and find ways to stay relevant despite decades of state policies aimed at its eradication. There has been a slow but clear shift in the state's valuation of what midwives can do for Mexico, such that even as some state representatives purportedly support some kinds of midwifery as a way to address some kinds of health issues, the trend has been to increasingly relegate midwives to the margins of health-care services. Why has it not disappeared completely? Why do midwifery schools continue to open nationwide, and midwives increasingly have the ear of politicians? Why are young women studying midwifery, and why are state clinics hiring them? The story of how midwives have been made to matter—and how midwives make themselves matter—is one that sits at the intersection of global health policies, national ideas about development and modernity, and the grassroots politics of small pockets of activists and practitioners who have found a way to insert the humanization of birth into the national agenda in such a way that the state cannot say no. This is the story that I tell in this book, through the midwives, educators, activists, and politicians who are shaping modern Mexican midwifery today.

All those years ago in my early days of following midwives around Mexico, however, I had no sense of how Juana's ability to acquire Pitocin, the patients' choices to go to village midwives against doctors' orders, or the concerns raised in the midwifery conference all related to bigger global and national debates. I saw the midwives I was meeting and learning from as practitioners, offering services to those who sought them out. I also did not see how precarious the fact of their existence was, nor did I understand the politics playing out behind the scenes that were to shape their future possibilities. It was through in-depth, ethnographic fieldwork that I learned how today's midwifery makes sense both in terms of the history of women's health in Mexico and contemporary understandings of how women's health outcomes fit into state visions for development and modernization. And I began to see midwives as more than just health-care providers; the work they do is about more than helping individual women manage pregnancy and birth. At a time when many of Mexico's most marginal populations continue to face high maternal mortality ratios, have difficulty accessing health care, receive sub-par medical treatment when they do receive it, and suffer the impacts of rampant obstetric violence, midwives present an alternative that promises to make an impact nationwide if given the chance. Further, their work extends beyond their interactions with patients. How midwives learn, where they practice, and how they interface with the state medical system are all questions with deep implications for the future of women's health in a country that is struggling to meet key development goals.[1]

In the chapters that follow, I look at how very different midwives and midwifery schools in Mexico are approaching the question of what midwives should know and do in Mexico today. I focus on midwifery education because it was through the schools' curricula, classroom discussions, and everyday transitions of students into practitioners that I was able to observe many aspects of what midwifery is becoming in Mexico today. Each of these schools tells us something distinct about how women's bodies are affected by processes of development and the spread of biomedicine into marginalized communities, and each offers a corrective that brings to light interconnected forces preventing women from attaining what the midwives all agree they should have as a basic right: dignified and humane treatment and access to trained professionals throughout their reproductive lives. Of course, midwifery in Mexico is nothing new; indeed, its changing roles and relationships with the Mexican state set the stage for the shape it has taken today (the next chapter will provide this historical context). Yet the midwifery of Mexico—and indeed, the world—is also not (only) old. To see it as a remnant of Mexico's traditional past is both ungenerous to the work contemporary midwives do and causes us to miss the point: that midwives— as they operate in spaces that deal in life and death, women and the healthcare system, citizenship and personhood—are working on modern bodies, in modern times, shaped by modern problems, and using the knowledge and resources made available by modern circuits.

Anthropologists have long described the impossibility of unlinking the local and the global, the particular and the universal, and the individual and the collective (Van Hollen 2011). This book adds to these revelations, in so much as it reveals the interconnectedness of the work midwives do with the worlds with which they interact, but it does not lead up to the global/local connection as an argument. Rather, I begin with the recognition that this connection is inevitably and inextricably present, and I move on from there. By the time I began working with midwives in Mexico in 2002, the internet was making connections between practitioners and access to resources increasingly practical and possible and necessary. By the time I began conducting the research for this book, some seven years later, social media was rapidly changing the pace by which midwives were connecting to each other, exchanging information, and organizing themselves. But before that, there were books—dog-eared copies of *Donde no hay doctor* (Werner 1980; Where there is no doctor), or Ina May Gaskin's (2002) *Spiritual Midwifery*—that I found on the shelves in midwives' homes and birth centers across Mexico that had clearly made the rounds for decades. And before that, there was word of mouth. Remedies passed through hands and moved through countries in suitcases and pockets; seeds traveled through the air or found new soil with colonial expansion (the *cardo santo* I helped Elena search for in the mountains of Oaxaca, for example, was written about by Shakespeare and was held dear in the European Middle Ages[2]). Global networks of knowledge and things are not new, and this book is not about tracing them or proving their existence.

This book is about how midwives working on the front lines of women's health in Mexico navigate their professions from this place of global connection. Specifically, it tells the story of how midwives are strategically navigating the changing global discourse around women's health to both strengthen their professional authority and improve health outcomes for their patients and communities. I show here the careful work that is done from this middle space that midwives occupy, and I argue that midwives simultaneously act *with* and push back *against* the Mexican state and global development initiatives as they push forward their own agendas.[3] As such, I position this book as an ethnography of what others have called "articulation" (Choy 2011) or the moments of "friction" (Tsing 2005). As Anna Tsing has argued, though, these terms do not reference a place of stagnation but rather a generative space. Through hard work, friction, and stickiness, things get done. As the midwives work with and against the infrastructures, ideas, technologies, attitudes, and assumptions of global health policies and interventions, they move things forward, ever pushing against the grindingly slow gears of bureaucracy and oppression. They do global health, but as they do it, they reshape it and make it their own.

On "Doing" Global Health

A couple of years ago, I attended a conference produced by and for nursing students at a nearby university where I was invited to speak about my research in Mexico. The keynote speaker was a nurse herself, who had spent many of her vacation days over the past decade traveling to poor countries on medical service trips to provide care to marginalized populations. As she told story after story of the extreme poverty she had witnessed, the gratitude patients expressed to her, and her own conflicted feelings of accomplishment and guilt over doing this work, she kept referring to what she did as "doing global health"—as in, "I did global health in Haiti, and then in Cuba, and then in Kenya." She quoted medical anthropologist and physician Paul Farmer (co-founder of Partners in Health) and showed images on the screen of children smiling at the camera in Haiti, Cuba, and Kenya. The students in the audience were enthralled, and inspired, and told me later that they, too, wanted to "do global health."

As an anthropologist, I was confused by the use of the term in this way. To me, global health was something to critically examine, not to "do." It referenced a sort of conceptual network of governments, NGOs, academics, and policies that is impossible to untangle but that becomes crystalized through products like the United Nations' Millennium Development Goals (MDGs) or the World Health Organization's Reports. Global health as a noun could be seen as a machine that takes in expert knowledge, demands numbers, and produces reports and policies for dispersal and implementation. So, when the speaker at the nursing conference said she was *doing* global health, I took notice.

As I have thought about the midwives I work with, I have sometimes come to think of them as "doing" global health as well, albeit in a very different way. For them, this is their daily life's work—hard and sometimes dangerous work; it is not something they do on vacation. But perhaps what the speaker shares with the midwives is that the work they are all doing responds to and reinforms how global health is addressed. Viewed this way, there is a hopeful undercurrent to this book: if midwives are part of the global health process, then they have the potential to change it. In the chapters that follow, I examine what midwives want changed and how they are positioning themselves to be the ones to make that change happen.

Global Health and Midwifery

What do I mean by global health in this context? First, what I do not mean: when Juana reaches for the drug Pitocin, or when Elena uses a European plant from the Middle Ages, they are not *doing* global health. These are examples of global connectedness, which may surprise and sometimes confound us in their unexpectedness. They are useful. They call our attention to places where something new is happening, or has happened in the past, and that has changed what we may have thought of as unchanging (e.g., midwifery). In paying attention to these places, we might start to unravel routes of knowledge and practice and to question our assumptions about where things come from.

Global health encompasses these dynamic places but does not value them. Global health values universals, not quirky local manifestations or improvisations. Yet the universal goals of global health policies cannot exist without the local to root them in reality. Global health is a concept, a network, a field of view that determines the stakes and sets the course of action for countries, states, and localities to adopt and follow, with the aim of achieving universal outcomes—low maternal mortality ratios, clean water, access to contraception, etc. Without the feedback of data from these places, there is no global health to *do*. Yet what data counts, how it gets interpreted, and how global health policies come to matter are not apolitical. Indeed, as Timothy Choy (2005) argues, what is understood as particular and universal are concepts created through (not prior to) political processes. The quest to achieve universals is a product itself of modern capitalism (Tsing 2005). In Chapter 2, I examine how the quest for universals led to the establishment of the Millennium Development Goals, and specifically the goal for reducing maternal mortality (referred to as MDG5). MDG5 is an example of how global health conceptualizes health problems and sets global goals for countries to achieve. I show how such problems and goals can both miss the mark and sometimes create opportunities for surprising new interventions and approaches to care.

Two important observations about global health approaches and interventions are that, in their quest for universality, they do not account for everyone and for all relevant health issues, and they do not address underlying structural problems. Anthropologists have long documented the mismatch between policies developed on an international scale and their local interpretations and manifestations (Justice 1987, 1989). Despite goals of reaching those who need help the most, it is often those who need the most who are the most difficult to reach. As João Biehl and Adriana Petryna write, global health interventions tend to "leave people behind, not only by limiting access to the services provided, but also by producing a parallel system of care and governance that undermines other avenues for care that might take into account broader systemic factors" (2013, 135). Technical and medical interventions cannot help those who cannot get to distribution sites because of lack of transportation or bad roads, for example, yet these interventions attract funders because of their seeming simplicity. Critics of these kinds of projects "have argued that such an emphasis on technical approaches ignores the more fundamental sources of suffering in developing countries—the living conditions of the world's poor" (Lakoff 2010, 67).

But even when those designing and distributing these kinds of interventions recognize the underlying poverty as the ultimate source of suffering, the question seems to be, what are they to do about it?

Complicated tensions between global health priorities and health interventions are, of course, not limited to the realm of childbirth or to the Mexican context. Indeed, Whitney Duncan's (2017) work on mental-health practice in Oaxaca, Mexico, illustrates how preoccupations with culture or cultural responses to modernization and globalization shape interventions. This takes the pressure off the state to invest in more meaningful and longer-lasting structural reform or to address underlying inequalities that are arguably more clearly to blame. Duncan says that when culture then becomes causally linked to poor health outcomes, "notions of culture are co-constructed with notions of modernity in ways that exculpate the state and shift responsibility to putatively 'cultural' citizens" (2017, 37). Dána-Ain Davis's (2019) work on premature birth among Black women in the United States similarly argues that interventions do not get at the root causes of poor health outcomes; for Davis, racist legacies pervade bodies in ways that resist public health interventions. Davis argues, then, that "interventions are unable to address racism . . . charts showing racial disparities do not address racism; health promotion campaigns focused on patients' behaviors and habits do not address racism" (206). Thus, interventions (often designed on a global scale to be implemented in diverse settings) are doomed to be ineffectual if they cannot get at the root causes of inequalities in health care or if they lay blame on individuals or "culture" for poor health outcomes.

This is where the midwives come into this story. They have seen how the global health perspective (represented by groups such as the UN, UNFPA, the MacArthur Foundation, etc.) has settled on a vision for what is wrong with women's health in what get called "developing regions," including Mexico. In this vision, women's health is synonymous with maternal health, and maternal mortality is frequently the ultimate indicator of development within maternal health. For Mexico to achieve the goals set forth by global health initiatives, it must reduce the number of women who die during or soon after childbirth to what is established as an acceptable number. The midwives I work with all agree, of course, that women should not die because of childbirth—the legitimacy of this goal is never contested. Yet they argue that maternal death is not the only concern facing women in Mexico and that, indeed, it is a symptom of many other structural issues that affect women's health in myriad ways. They argue that women's health in Mexico has become conditional to certain kinds of outcomes. The conditional nature of maternal health care in Mexico has rendered women vulnerable to the myopic goals of global health approaches as interpreted through national health-care policies and programs. These policies and programs are accountable to numerical targets, outcomes that do not care so much about the quality of care or about women's desires.

Ethnographic methods are well suited to bring attention to the qualitative aspects of women's health care under such conditions. They also allow us to see how individual experiences, desires, and outcomes in health are related to conversations and interventions at local, national, and global levels. As João Biehl and Adriana Petryna write, ethnography allows for the sort of telescoping of scale that "lays bare how interventions are woven into larger spheres of political economy and points to the impact of structural and economic factors on treatment and disease" (2013, 136). On the other hand, they continue, it has the potential to lead to actionable ideas; by accounting for deeper connections and widening the field of view beyond a search for prescribed measures (like maternal mortality data), "new ways of looking at care and accountability might result" (136). Cecilia Van Hollen (2003), for example, shows through ethnographic engagement how global development's impacts on women's experiences of childbirth and maternity in India are not always what development agencies have in mind.

In building claims about how global health approaches to maternal health are interpreted and manifested in Mexico, I recognize that I am unable to capture the complete nature of "global health"—it is too big. Yet, as a concept, it was present in all of my interactions: it shaped them, and it provided vocabulary from which midwives, doctors, and policymakers alike could draw. I find Anna Tsing's approach to thinking about the global useful. Tsing suggests that we examine the global by looking at the moments of friction, the "zones of awkward engagement, where words mean something different across a divide even as people agree to speak" (2005, xi). Throughout this book I encounter such differences. Sometimes people are knowingly strategic in their use of terms and ideas in unexpected ways—as when midwives use language around maternal mortality reduction as a way to argue for the validity of their profession—but other times, we see how awkward engagements lead to poor outcomes—as when the global push to get women into hospitals leaves some women left literally outside.

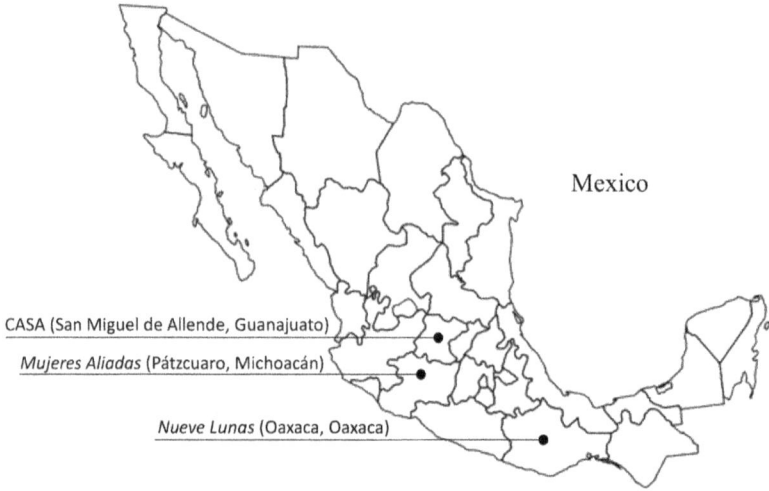

Mexico

CASA (San Miguel de Allende, Guanajuato)

Mujeres Aliadas (Pátzcuaro, Michoacán)

Nueve Lunas (Oaxaca, Oaxaca)

FIGURE 2: Map of Mexico with primary research sites.

Sites and Methods

The research for this book was conducted over seventeen months between 2009 and 2012. Follow-up interviews were conducted over the next few years, and I remained in touch with many of my informants throughout the intervening years through social media and email. I have visited them in person as well. I was based in the town of San Miguel de Allende, Guanajuato, in colonial central Mexico, and spent the majority of my time there at CASA's midwifery clinic and school. This was the city where I had originally come to learn about Mexico's professional midwives, and it made sense as a research base because of CASA's role in the changing landscape of the midwifery profession. The two other schools where I spent time and that are featured in this book, Mujeres Aliadas (Allied Women) in Pátzcuaro, Michoacán, and Nueve Lunas (Nine Moons—a reference to the months of pregnancy) in Oaxaca City, Oaxaca, had opened in the years since I first began working with Mexican midwives (Figure 2 shows where the schools are located in Mexico). They were also struggling to become part of the official education and health-care system and to gain recognition for their own models of teaching and practice, which differed significantly from CASA's. It took me years to appreciate many of the differences between these schools; I recognize that, for readers, such distinctions will certainly blur throughout this

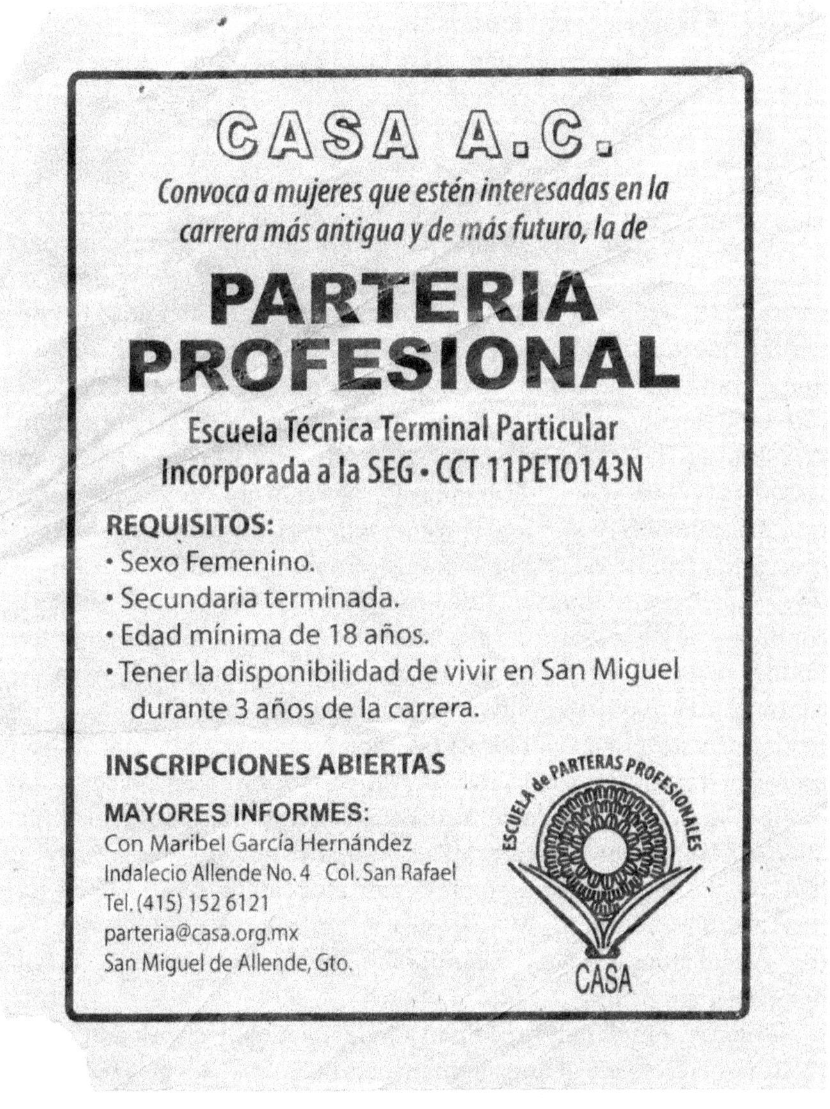

FIGURE 3: Recruitment advertisement for CASA midwifery school.

book. I thus offer below my brief summary of each school's history, approach, and student population so that readers may return here for a quick reminder when I reference them in the following chapters. In addition, I offer short profiles of three students from each of the schools during the time I was conducting research; while I wish I could tell all of their diverse stories here, these brief details give a glimpse of the range of backgrounds, experiences, and aspirations of contemporary Mexican midwifery students (see the sidebars in the next sections).

CASA

CASA began in 1981 first as a sexual health education site and contraception provider. Its midwifery school was opened in 1997 and was considered the first professional midwifery program of its kind.[4] Founder Nadine Goodman had begun the school upon the requests of local traditional midwives (including the same Doña Guadalupe from the Prologue) who wanted consistent, formal training that the state was not offering.[5] From the start, CASA worked with the state education and health-care systems to create an institutionalized program whose graduates' careers would be officially recognized and compensated. Students were recruited specifically from rural and Indigenous communities nationwide (though they came from all kinds of cities and towns and some even from other countries) and had only to be eighteen years old and to have completed middle school to attend CASA; the goal was for them to return to their communities to practice once they completed the program.[6] Figure 3 is a recruitment advertisement for CASA's schools that illustrates these simple prerequisites. Interestingly, it calls at the top for women who "are interested in the oldest and most futuristic career, professional midwifery." Most students received nearly full scholarships at CASA so that they only had to pay about six hundred Mexican pesos (at the time, around forty-five US dollars) a month. While this was still a hardship for many (who took on side jobs or relied on family support), the scholarships certainly helped a great deal.

Students completed three intensive years of coursework and clinical rotations in biomedical and alternative healing practices at CASA's maternity hospital and in the local public hospital. They also completed annual homestays with traditional midwives and, like other health professionals, a year of social service upon graduation. Their training culminated in a terminal, "technical" level degree in professional midwifery that was recognized by the federal government and allowed them to get work and a steady salary in government clinics and hospitals.[7]

Despite Nadine's goals to provide quality training in midwifery, offer educational opportunities that lead to stable careers, and improve women's health

Three Students from CASA

Alma's central concern as she finished her last year at CASA was how to find balance. She described how disorienting it could be, learning one week from a traditional midwife and the next from a doctor in the hospital during clinical rotations, but she also sought balance between the groups of midwives she was slowly coming to know as she got more involved in the national midwifery scene. She did not like debates over who counted as a "real" midwife. She saw the value in traditional midwifery knowledge and methods, but she had also witnessed the skills she had learned in the hospital being used to save a woman's life. She said her dream job would be to work in the city of Guanajuato but that she would also consider returning to CASA to teach someday.

Sara was a first-year student at CASA. She came from a community near the city San Luis Potosí, about a two-hour drive north of the school, where her parents lived and took care of her two-year-old son. They brought her son to see her, or she went there to visit him when she could, which she said was quite hard on them all. However, she thought this difficult time would be worth it in the end, when she returned home to her community to help people there. "We have no local doctor, no health-care options in my community," she explained. As a licensed midwife, she would eventually be able to bring a needed skill to the whole region. She commented that "it seems hard to imagine that things will change with just one or two people, but I have to believe we can make a difference."

Natalia was one of a few Guatemalan students who came to CASA to train as professional midwives with the plan of returning to Guatemala and hopefully, someday, starting a similar program there. She was one of nine children who grew up with her family three hours outside of Guatemala City on a coffee plantation. Back home, she had been studying to enter into university, but then she found out about this program and decided to come. She was initially not sure whether she had made the right choice, but then she saw her first birth and exclaimed, "Eso es lo mío!" (This is my thing!). In her final year at CASA, she felt that she had learned so much. She had a job lined up in Guatemala upon graduation but was considering staying in Mexico for a while first; while at CASA, she had the opportunity to travel all over the country, and she loved getting to learn about new places.

conditions nationwide, CASA's vision was not without local opposition. From the beginning, many local physicians and politicians loudly opposed CASA's efforts to train professional midwives. Margot, who graduated in CASA's first generation of professional midwives, described to me how the doctors in town marched against CASA on the day that it opened (since that time, many doctors and politicians have come to support CASA and even teach there). While on the one hand, midwives were seen as unnecessary or even dangerous, on the other hand, CASA received criticism because of its emphasis on reproductive health in one of the most conservative states in Mexico.[8]

I chose CASA as my primary field site both because of its status as an established program that was already entrenched in the state and national healthcare and education systems and because of my own historical connection to it. I had first come to CASA in 2002 as an intern, and between 2002 and 2007 I worked as a volunteer, translator, and workshop teacher there intermittently. My own daughter was born at CASA in 2006 with one of the founding midwives on staff at the time—an experience that certainly contributes to my interest in and reflections on this research (and on which I reflect in the Prologue). The relationships that I made during those early years working with CASA midwives and staff were invaluable when I returned to conduct my research. Because I already had an in-depth knowledge of CASA's programs, I was able to determine that the current pressing concerns faced by CASA and its midwives had to do with the future of midwifery education in Mexico and the role of "professional" midwives in the national health-care system. That intimate knowledge, gained over many years, proved a solid place to start. As Sandra Harding argues, "there are important resources for the production of knowledge to be found in starting off research projects from issues arising in women's lives rather than only from the dominant androcentric conceptual frameworks of the disciplines and the larger social order" (1998, 149). When I returned to the field and re-established contact with my midwife friends, I was asked directly to help them by looking at the bigger historical and geographical picture of midwifery in Mexico today. Further, midwives stressed to me that CASA was struggling to maintain and increase its authority within the health-care system—and quickly noted that it was no longer the only outspoken midwifery school in the country. Two newer schools (described below) offered striking alternatives to what CASA had been doing. As I learned about them, it became clear that, while all of the schools' founders and students shared a common view that midwifery could improve women's health in Mexico, there were sharply divergent notions about how midwives should learn and what their relationship to the state should be.

MUJERES ALIADAS

Mujeres Aliadas, founded by an American nurse midwife from Chicago whom I call Diana, also offered its students three years of training in biomedical and alternative medical practices. It was originally focused on training local nurses, with the goal of sending them back to their nearby communities to offer quality maternal health care. According to the students I surveyed

Three Students from Mujeres Aliadas

Mariana was from a small town near Mujeres Aliadas. She was thirty-six years old, had three children, and had been married since she was sixteen. She entered this program without really knowing what professional midwifery was but said that she started realizing how much more information and better care women in her region needed. Now, she said, "I want to change how women are treated and teach women about their rights and their bodies."

Victoria was studying nursing at the same time as completing this program. She said that many young women in her village were getting pregnant, and she wanted to help them and to prevent unwanted pregnancies in general. As a nursing student, she had been observing how poorly women were treated in hospitals, and she wanted to change that as well, through providing better care and educating women. "I want to help women to value their bodies," she said, "by explaining everything about their bodies to them so that they know what is happening."

Gabriela was thirty-seven years old and came from a small town a short distance from Mujeres Aliadas. She trained as a nurse but never got to work as one. Instead, she had worked for years assisting her traditional midwife grandmother. Together, they attended women with all kinds of issues, using plants as their primary medicinal source. Gabriela said that when she heard about the program at Mujeres Aliadas, "I felt like I'd been waiting for it for years!" But she did note that the program thus far had been very different from traditional midwifery as she knew it.

there, most had never had hands-on experience with women in labor before beginning the program, although they all had clinical experience as nurses. More recently, Mujeres Aliadas has received the same national government recognition CASA fought to create and has expanded its entrance requirements to allow students who are not yet nurses (but who must have at least a high-school diploma, in contrast to CASA's middle-school requirement). I contacted the founders of Mujeres Aliadas and was able to visit their school twice to observe in the classroom, conduct a survey and interviews with their students, and talk many times with their administrators.

NUEVE LUNAS

Nueve Lunas was the most distinct of the three schools. During my time in Mexico before graduate school, I had also lived and worked with midwives in Oaxaca; there, I met the women who would go on to become the school's founders, so I was later able to re-establish contact with them for

Three Students from Nueve Lunas

Paula came to Nueve Lunas in part because of her grandmother and in part because she had been interested in studying medicine. Her grandmother helped pregnant women by giving them prenatal massages, or sobadas, to help position the baby for labor. Paula grew up following her grandmother around as she massaged pregnant women and helped them through their pregnancy-related discomforts with herbs, mostly in the form of teas.

Catalina was from a small town near the coast, about a six-hour drive from the Nueve Lunas school. She said that she felt she needed to come take this training, as there were no more midwives left in her region. The women there did not like going to give birth in the clinics because they were treated so badly, but then there was nobody else with the knowledge and skills to help them. "I have seen cases where babies die," she said, "because they couldn't get good care." She said that some women would find their way to a clinic because of financial incentives, but that nobody wanted to go there because of how badly they were treated.

María José was from a neighborhood just outside of Oaxaca City and came from a family of midwives. Her mother was a traditional midwife, and her sister went through the first generation of the Nueve Lunas program. María José's dream had always been to become a midwife as well. When she was growing up, she used to always try to help her mother, but her mother always told her to just keep going to school, to keep studying before trying to start working. Then one day, her mother let María José watch a birth, and she was even more convinced that she needed to do this work. Her mother used traditional medicines such as plants, never allopathic remedies.

this research. Nueve Lunas was also a three-year program that called its graduates "autonomous midwives" or "professional midwives," despite not following the same curricula as CASA or Mujeres Aliadas (and despite its graduates being unable to achieve the federally recognized licensure). The school aimed to train women who would carry on the local traditions and practices of the midwives in their own villages, while also equipping graduates with internationally recognized best practices in midwifery. Students came together for one week a month in Oaxaca City to do workshops based on international norms for midwifery practice, but the rest of the time they were on their own, apprenticing with their local traditional midwives. While Nueve Lunas continues to actively offer training, the state recently made them take down the school's website because their teachers did not hold state-recognized credentials (Atkin et al. 2017). I visited Nueve Lunas to interview students, teachers, and administrators during February 2012.

An overarching finding was that each of these three schools considered their graduates "professional" midwives (*parteras profesionales*), even if the term itself was debated endlessly on the basis of differing opinions on what constitutes a professional—does a professional need a high-school degree? A college degree? Official government recognition? Yet despite such debates, the shared image of a new kind of professional midwife who was able to address Mexico's needs through a compassionate, educated, and evidence-based approach to women's health linked all these schools.

Another shared feature across these schools was the contradictory nature of their geographic locations. On the one hand, each of these schools was located in a picturesque, colonial city with plenty of tourists and foreign expatriates coming through or settling nearby. This meant that there was money flowing through these regions and volunteers on hand. Yet each place also, importantly, mapped onto a region of high maternal mortality; the schools' states of Michoacán, Oaxaca, and Guanajuato all are listed in the top half of Mexican states for maternal deaths (OMM 2019). The fact that such popular tourist and expat locations, with such rich cultural history, are also in states with extreme poverty and economic inequality (Aguilar Ortega 2019) meant that the schools, their administrators, and their students all had to learn to navigate multiple worlds as they advocated for midwifery's value.

My own positionality in these spaces is not uncomplicated, as is often the case during ethnographic research. As a foreigner, I blended into the tourist and expat crowds but stood out while observing in classrooms or clinics. Yet the fact of my own daughter's birth with one of the well-known midwives at CASA, my years spent living and working in Mexico prior to conducting my research, and my integration into regular life as a single parent doing regular parenting things all helped me forge trusting relationships that I otherwise might not have.

Throughout my fieldwork, I examined Mexican midwifery education on multiple levels and in multiple settings through participant observation in classrooms and student presentations, clinical rotations and home visits, administrative and political meetings, and national and international midwifery conferences. During observations, I kept thorough hand-written field notes and typed them up twice a week in order to add reflections and note emergent themes that could later be used in interviews. Only during planned and more formal interviews was a recording device used; I wanted to keep my observations casual, as I felt that bringing a computer or recorder into classes or talks would be obtrusive in settings where most students took handwritten notes. I wanted to see how midwives were learning and how that training was translating into practice and being debated among midwives, administrators, and politicians across Mexico. Because I spent the majority of my time at CASA, I was able to watch students progress throughout their training and into their early careers. I became close with many students and staff, and our conversations outside CASA enriched my understanding of their achievements, struggles, and goals. At Mujeres Aliadas and Nueve Lunas, I observed and spoke with students during class and break times, and I socialized with them outside school to get to know more about their lives and aspirations.

While in classroom settings at each site, I observed regular educational activities and lessons with midwifery students of all years in the programs and assisted midwifery professors when requested. During class breaks, I talked with students and teachers about their reactions to class materials. I took notes on class lessons, as well as on students' questions, reactions, and doubts about materials. Classroom time was also when administrators occasionally gave talks to students about concerns facing midwifery in Mexico today, which thus provided me the opportunity to witness students learning about these issues. During my time conducting participant observations at the CASA clinic, I observed routine encounters with midwives, doctors, and students. These consisted mostly of prenatal and postnatal exams, family planning visits, and women's health checkups, but they also included births in clinical and home settings. My attention in these clinical encounters was on the educational process and the relationships between students, among students and teachers (staff midwives), and among students and patients; I was not studying the patients themselves. However, due to the potentially sensitive nature of many of the clinical encounters, I obtained verbal consent from all patients before entering the room for observations.

While I informally spoke with and observed a total of sixty-five midwifery students across the three school sites, I conducted more focused, semi-structured interviews with a subset of twenty students; these students reflected the diverse backgrounds of the larger student midwife population and came from different programs and years within those programs. I conducted semi-structured interviews with eleven practicing midwives (working at the three schools or involved in national debates over standardization), fifteen school administrators, and four doctors. With the majority of those interviewed, various follow-up interviews occurred throughout the field-work period. Additionally, I administered a survey to thirty-eight midwifery students from CASA and Mujeres Aliadas schools, which examined students' career goals and understandings about the current and future roles of midwives in the Mexican health-care system. This survey also included a section asking students to draw pictures of what birth looked like in the hospitals and what their ideal birth with a midwife would look like. By analyzing these images, survey responses, detailed interview transcripts, and field notes, I began to understand Mexican midwifery education from various perspectives and angles. All participants who were interviewed gave verbal consent in accordance with my university's IRB requirements, and most have been given pseudonyms; political figures quoted during public conferences and events, however, retain their real names.

While patients and their families appear in this book, they were not the focus of my research, and therefore their stories are not highlighted here. I struggled with the question of whether I should seek IRB approval to interview patients as well. Ultimately, I decided that, despite the clear importance of their perspectives on midwifery and health care, this project was more specifically about the midwives and their schools. I wanted to focus on their work and how they made sense of it, as well as their interactions with the state and their professional struggles and aspirations. Their patients were ever present—whether in the exam rooms, at a home birth, or evoked in the classroom—but I was interested in how the midwives and their students interpreted patient needs, experiences, and health outcomes. I refer readers to other excellent recent work that thoughtfully includes women's stories in their own words, such as Davis's (2019) book on premature birth in the United States, Carson et al.'s (2017) article including the voices of multiple early-age mothers in Canada, Vania Smith-Oka's (2014, 2015; Smith-Oka and Rokhideh 2018) many publications on women's experiences with health care in Mexico, or Sarah Rubin's (2018) work on motherhood and poverty in South Africa.

In addition to my three primary school sites, I spent time at Luna Maya (Maya Moon) midwifery clinic and school in San Cristobal de las Casas, Chiapas, as well as the private home clinics of midwives located across Mexico. Those midwives whom I contacted but could not visit (because of distance) I was able to communicate with via email, telephone, and Skype. I attended a two-week-long training retreat in 2009 for midwives, doulas, and birth activists from across Mexico in the mountain town of Malinalco, a 2010 national midwifery conference in San Cristobal de las Casas, Chiapas, a 2012 forum on humanized birth in Mexico City, the first open meeting for the Mexican Midwifery Association in 2012, and many smaller, regional conferences, political meetings, and public events related to midwifery and women's health in Mexico. At all of these events, I was able to meet and talk with people who held stakes in the future of Mexican midwifery and opinions about how midwifery education should best be structured.

In each phase of research, I was concerned with how midwifery models of care were being shaped by notions of tradition, modernity, and development. These are all loaded and potentially troubling terms. I grapple with shifting definitions and uses for "tradition," resisting the pull to contrast it with modernity or development. Modernity was a concept equally difficult to pin down but which pervaded local and national discussions of what the Mexican health-care system needed; its definitions and the ramifications of the policies it motivates have formed a central concern among scholars of Mexico (such as Néstor García Canclini, Claudio Lomnitz, and Octavio Paz). Beatriz Reyes-Foster draws on such scholarship in her own work on psychiatry in Mexico, where she finds that "the Mexican state's obsession with becoming *modern* figures prominently"; yet modernity in Mexico must always be evaluated, she reminds us, in relationship with its ever present, dark counterpart: coloniality (2018, 12). Similarly, this obsession permeates the framing of this book. Thus, this work seeks not only to address the specific situation of midwives in Mexico, but also to inform our understanding of how debates of modernity in developing regions contribute to health-care practices and, ultimately, health outcomes. Similarly, the term "development" carries distinct meanings at local, national, and global registers and is not always used in a uniform way. This is a term that many activists, scholars, and even the World Bank have been wary of because of its lack of specificity and because of the potentially offensive implications of the term (Khokhar and Serajuddin 2015), but it is still largely used among global health programs. While I find the concept highly problematic, I use it here because of its continued presence in conversations about policies and interventions related to women's health in Mexico and beyond.

There has been much written about midwifery in Mexico, and I hope that this book can add to the literature in unique ways. Brigitte Jordan's (1978) *Birth in Four Cultures*, which she researched in part in Yucatán, Mexico, set the stage for the ethnographic study of knowledge and authority in birth. Robbie Davis-Floyd continued Jordan's legacy and has written specifically about the advent of professional midwifery and the various types of midwifery models in Mexico and beyond, alone and in various important collaborations that have added to our understanding of how such models diverge and what can be learned from them (see, e.g., Davis-Floyd [2001a, 2001b, and 2005]; Davis-Floyd, Pigg, and Cosminsky [2001]; Benoit and Davis-Floyd [2004]). Davis-Floyd (2001a) suggests that the relatively new professional midwives (whom she terms "postmodern midwives") draw smartly from tools of "modernity" while recasting traditional knowledge as valuable and possibly patriotic. The image that Davis-Floyd paints of the postmodern midwife suggests an interesting set of divisions: First is the division between the pre-modern midwife—who is associated with the nation's undeveloped past, with poor training and poor settings—and the modern physician, who is associated with development, Westernization, and technical expertise. Second is the division between the modern physician—who gets reframed as oppressive and limited by biomedical knowledge—and the postmodern midwife—who emerges as the ideal balance between past and future, biomedicine and its alternatives, women and the health-care industry. I have found this conceptualization a helpful starting place from which to think about professional midwives as working within, around, and through such divisions.

More recently, Rosalynn A. Vega has written an analysis of midwifery in Mexico that draws on her extensive ethnographic research, much of it overlapping geographically and temporally with my own. Vega's central concern is with how "traditional Mexican midwifery is transformed into a series of commodified practices that are then marketed in other countries, and how humanized-birth techniques originating in the Global North are combined with 'traditional' methods through a New Age logic that confounds Euro-American notions of chronology and progress" (2018, 152). She takes a critical view of professional midwifery in Mexico, linking it to the humanization of birth movement, which, she argues, "inadvertently commodifies Indigenous culture in symbolically cannibalistic ways" (24). My arguments depart from Vega's in that, while I agree that we should pay attention to the treatment of traditional midwives, I am more interested in the ways that *both* professional and traditional midwives strategically and pragmatically select from the methods available to them to treat the women they can under the best circumstances they can manage. Further, I show here how efforts to humanize birth (through, for example, fighting against obstetric violence or advocating for changes to hospital-based obstetric care) are not categorically elitist (though Vega offers examples of how this can sometimes be the case) but are instead part of a shared goal across types of midwives to improve the quality of care for all women.

Mounia El Kotni (2016) and Veronica Miranda (2017) have also written recent work about midwifery in Mexico that critically examines relationships between traditional midwives and the state. Indeed, the three of us have collectively considered the ways that different types of midwives across Mexico learn their craft and conceptualize their careers from spaces of marginalization (Dixon, El Kotni, and Miranda 2019). In recognizing different levels of access and support for different kinds of midwives, El Kotni brings up important questions that echo Vega's concerns, as she notes that in Chiapas, some professional midwives "are out of reach for most of the women covered by Seguro Popular [Popular Health Insurance program] and mostly cater to middle- and upper-class women" (2018, 66). This concern underscores the reality that, if professional midwifery and the humanized treatment it proposes are to become valid options for all women, there will need to be large-scale integration with the existing health-care system. What that should look like, however, is not an easy question to answer.

Framing Concepts

WORKING "WITH AND AGAINST"

Global development initiatives have begun to frame midwives as useful tools in reaching marginalized populations and improving maternal health outcomes, an attitude that has filtered down to the national level across Mexico and, in many ways, lies beneath midwives' current resurgence in acceptance. As midwives join Mexico's struggle to reach development goals like maternal mortality reduction, they are not always in easy partnership with the state. When they step into hospital maternity wards and don scrubs and surgical gloves, midwives confront conflicting notions of care and approaches to women. Midwifery students, trained in a range of educational models across Mexico, are working alongside biomedical practitioners in state institutions, working with politicians to ensure their legitimacy, and participating in national conversations about women's health.

However, as they work strategically alongside the state, midwives are also maintaining momentum in activist movements to address gender-based inequalities affecting women's health and lives. Their unique insider/outsider position affords them a critical vantage point from which to speak to the failures of development policies in women's health, the lack of holistic women's health care, and the prevalence of what they call obstetric violence within biomedical institutions. Midwives must strategically maneuver the tensions that arise from being simultaneously *with* the institutions that afford them authority and the ability to practice and *against* the practices and attitudes they witness therein. I borrow Michelle Murphy's (2017) idea of working or living "with and against" to describe the position that midwives find themselves in, which can be both oppressively confining and surprisingly generative. While for Murphy, this push-pull relationship is elaborated in terms of technoscientific and chemical entanglements that she lives within as she pushes back against them, I argue that Mexican midwifery must be understood as already in relationship with the very state systems that it is critiquing. The very term "midwife" (whose name, in English, comes from the words "with woman"), holds within it an orientation that prioritizes the women being served, a perspective that midwives feel is absent in the health-care system they are trying to work within and alongside, which therefore compels action and reaction.

Throughout this book I attempt to accurately describe the push-pull relationship that characterizes my understanding of Mexican midwifery during a time of modernization and development: the midwives need the state—they depend on state institutions for licensure, salaries in some cases, certificates, and occasional opportunities for work—but they are also some of the strongest critics of the practices employed in state facilities. Midwives in Mexico work both with and against the Mexican state as they strive to improve women's health experiences and outcomes. In this position, they have to navigate the tensions they feel as they witness entrenched social inequalities, structural failures, and legacies of misogyny and colonialism colliding with urgent efforts to improve women's health.

I examine these tensions from the point of view of the midwives and midwifery students who are working on the front lines, within the intersection of global development policies, national projects of modernization, and grassroots activism. I argue that the very trends inherent to modernization and development which long pushed midwives out of the system in the name of improving health for all are now creating space for midwives' reentry and the platform upon which midwives can craft nuanced, broadly reaching critiques of the way women's health is prioritized and addressed.

Central to my analysis is a recognition of the intersectional oppression felt by many of the women and communities midwives are trying to help—and indeed, felt by many of the midwives as well. In referencing Mexico's "poor" or "marginalized," the full weight of such oppression is not always reflected. Mexico is a country of economic extremes (home to many of the world's extremely rich and extremely poor). Recent studies show that income inequality in Mexico is high and increasing (del Castillo Negrete Rovira 2017). However, according to the World Bank (2019), Mexico is considered an upper-middle income economy (a category that puts it alongside countries including Sri Lanka, China, and Cuba). Yet this designation glosses over the vast discrepancies in countries like Mexico between the very rich and the very poor and erases distinctions between economic development in rural versus urban regions. Roldán et al. argue that such country-level categorization can "both conceal and erase extreme poverty in rural zones" (2017, 3). Despite its upper-middle income designation, much of Mexico continues to struggle economically.

The percentage of households living in moderate or extreme poverty is higher in rural regions than in urban regions; in cases of extreme poverty this difference was much more marked in rural areas, findings that have been linked to urbanization and international trade agreements such as NAFTA. This inequality plays out across segments of the population in compounding ways: three quarters of Mexico's Indigenous population (which itself makes up 10 percent of the national population) live in rural areas (Puyana and Murillo 2012).

Indigeneity brings more than economic inequality. Recent research has highlighted many significant forms of discrimination faced by Mexicans with darker skin tones, from educational to employment attainment (Monroy-Gómez-Franco, Vélez Grajales, and Yalonetzky 2018). While the racism that Indigenous people experience in Mexico and across Latin America may present differently than in places like the United States because of distinct colonial histories, the discrimination that Indigenous people experience in the health-care system in particular is a form of medical racism. Davis helpfully defines medical racism as "the ideas and practices that perpetuate racial hierarchies and compromise one's health or facilitate vulnerability to premature illness or death" (2019, 8). Mexico's deep divisions in access to care and health outcomes cannot be understood without an awareness of the ways that medical racism plays out among Indigenous populations, especially in matters of reproduction.

In addition to rurality and indigeneity, Mexico continues to reflect deep inequalities around gender. Gender violence affects women across the board: 66 percent of women over age fifteen have been victim to some form of violence (INEGI 2018), a point that has led Mexico to increasingly address issues of gender harassment, assault, and femicides. In Chapter 1, I examine more closely how gender inequalities intersect with rurality and indigeneity among outcomes in education and employment. For those women who are also Indigenous and/or live in rural regions of the country, the deck is stacked against them. This matters in important ways when we consider health-care services and health outcomes.

The Mexican health-care system struggles to provide care to all, and the areas where it has not been sufficient reflect and reinforce the inequalities described above. As Roldán et al. note, "The social polarization in Mexico . . . exposes extreme marginalization between the Indigenous and urban worlds and inequality of access to health services. The lack of public health service coverage most frequently occurs in Indigenous and rural localities" (2017, 10).

Throughout this book, in referencing efforts aimed at ameliorating these intersectional inequalities—efforts that originate from grassroots all the way to national and global spheres—I use the term "development." That is, I discuss the goals, policies, and practices being experimented with across Mexico as part of the project of global development, an idea that in turn evokes the idea that Mexico is itself develop*ing*. In recent years concerns have been raised about classifications of countries as "developed" or "developing"—terms for which the United Nations explicitly states there is no established definition (UN 2018). Projects and policies launched within the framing of development may sound unified in their virtuous goals but internally reflect conflicting and changeable power dynamics, agendas, and understandings about what could and should be done (Closser 2010; Justice 1989). Yet the terms continue to be used, even as they perhaps outlive their value, because they have found their way into policies and shaped the way global health targets have evolved. Indeed, despite the problems with this terminology (Khokhar and Serajuddin 2015), I suggest that Mexico's continuing classification by the United Nations as a "developing" country allows actors like the midwives in this book to frame their efforts within a vision for change and growth. Further, it allows them to back up their assertions of widespread health-care system failure in global classification.

AUTHENTICITY POLITICS AND CRITIQUES OF FOREIGN FOUNDERS

In discussing Mexican midwifery as engaged in a push-pull relationship with the Mexican state, I cannot ignore that the three midwifery schools examined here were themselves created out of a historically complicated position: that of transnational NGOs with foreign founders. CASA was co-founded by an American with a master's degree in public health. Mujeres Aliadas was co-founded by an American nurse midwife. Nueve Lunas was co-founded by an Italian midwife along with a Mexican midwife. While each school's founding also involved local, Mexican partners and was designed to meet specific local needs, they have all come under various levels of critique because of their foreign roots and influences.

While I disagree with the notion that traditional knowledge is fixed in time and geographic location (indeed, practitioners of "traditional" Mexican midwifery use a range of techniques that have origins beyond Mexico), I recognize that it is important to pay attention when foreigners make claims about how best to solve local problems, especially related to health. The past decade has seen a rise in critical anthropology of medical humanitarianism that has urged us to question the impacts of humanitarian work that imports funding and/or ideologies from global sources with their own diverse political or social commitments (Abramowitz and Panter-Brick 2015). The kind of medical humanitarianism we see today has increasingly shifted away from disaster relief and emergency aid toward more lasting interventions, like clinic building, such that it now "holds a prominent presence in international development, global health, human rights advocacy, and international peacekeeping and diplomacy" (Abramowitz and Panter-Brick 2015, 4).

Further, concerns over the expansion of what author Teju Cole (2012) has dubbed the "White Savior Industrial Complex" bring to light questions of what it means to do good, to not do harm, and to actually seek and use local input when designing programs meant to help people. Cole was referencing the proliferation of (usually white) foreigners intervening to "help" without first asking what kind of help—if any—people want (and frequently posting exuberantly about their experiences on social media). I do not think this particular analysis applies to the founders of midwifery schools in Mexico, but I agree that their positionality as foreigners with high education levels and relative levels of privilege merits critical discussion. That they were all able to begin successful education programs in Mexico is not only a product of their individual tenacity and skills (though that is certainly part of it), but it also reflects the intersecting histories of foreign aid, health care, development, and governance in Latin America and Mexico in particular.

The fact that the three midwifery schools profiled in this book are not state run makes sense if we look at this intersecting history. When CASA opened in 1981 and then started its school in 1997, it was one of thousands of NGOs popping up worldwide during that time (one estimate is that global NGOs increased from six to sixty thousand from 1990 to 1998; with that increase came billions of dollars of aid as well) (Schuller 2012). NGOs had been increasing steadily across Latin America since the late 1970s, bringing that aid money with them and taking on services not provided by the state (Elgar 2014, 362). This shift was tied to an increase in neoliberalism and supported the decentralization of the government (Richard 2009) but also reflected a lack of trust in state organizations, especially in the wake of the government's poor response to the 1982 debt crisis and the 1985 Mexico City earthquake (Mills 2010).

By the 1980s, the field of reproductive health rights advocacy began to see a proliferation of international aid and brought an increased presence of global organizations to Mexico, including USAID, Oxfam, International Planned Parenthood Federation, United Nations Population Fund (UNFPA), UNICEF, the W. K. Kellogg Foundation, as well as regional organizations such as the Pan American Health Organization (Atkin et al. 2017; Elgar 2014; Mills 2010). Many of these organizations have been involved over the years in the evaluation of midwifery education and practice in Mexico, often funding schools or related studies. The John D. and Catherine T. MacArthur Foundation, for example, has played a major role in researching and advocating for midwifery and women's reproductive health rights in Mexico for decades. In 2015, they invested seventeen million US dollars in grant funding to evaluate the state of professional midwifery in Mexico at that time and to develop strategies for making it a sustainable practice that could have a measurable impact on women's health outcomes (Atkin et al. 2019, 5).

It is important to note that national and local NGOs (not just international ones) were emerging across Mexico at this time as well; in 1992, the group GIRE (the Information Group on Reproductive Choice) was started out of the Mexican feminist movement, "with the mission and the vision of contributing to the recognition, respect, and guarantee of reproductive rights in Mexico" (GIRE 2012, 13; my translation). Mujeres Aliadas and Nueve Lunas came later, but their emergence is part of this broader trajectory of NGOs taking on reproductive health-care training and advocacy in Mexico.

Despite the public perception that NGOs circumvent complicated bureaucracies to do good, give voice to marginalized populations, and get real work done on the ground (that governments cannot or will not do), anthropologists have raised important questions about their monolithic status; ethnographic description has brought to light complex motivations that actors within such organizations may bring (Schuller 2012).

An important critique of NGOs and of humanitarian indicatives more broadly is that they may not be sustainable or scalable. As an anthropologist interested in underlying structural causes of inequality in health, I have thought critically about how the schools described here have struggled to make themselves sustainable by addressing those very causes, albeit in very different ways. For CASA, this has meant working with the state from the start and creating a scalable model for other states to take on as government projects (a process that few NGOs have managed to do) (Pick, Givaudan, and Reich 2008). For Mujeres Aliadas this has been about bringing holistic gynecological care into the midwifery training model and also achieving certification for their graduates to find paid work. For Nueve Lunas it has been about creating networks to retain and promote traditional midwifery knowledge while creating opportunities for practicing midwives. None of these claims to address underlying concerns guarantees that these organizations will prevail, but they indicate a desire to enact long-term change. Further, they represent what Pick, Givaudan, and Reich (2008) argue is the most effective work of NGOs: that of figuring out how to most effectively address issues that the government may want to address but may not have the resources or support to dedicate to the task.

While CASA and, to an extent, Mujeres Aliadas have sought to work directly with the state and national government to scale up their models for midwifery education, Nueve Lunas has been wary of such collaborations, concerned in part about the influence of state regulations on what they see as a necessarily and inherently flexible occupation. The differences expressed between the schools about whether or not to work with the state reflect a divide among Latin American feminists that dates back to the 1980s, between those who wanted to work with the state to create changes and those who wanted to remain autonomous (Elgar 2014, 352). For CASA founder Nadine, the "right" way to create lasting change was by changing the system; for some other midwives and school administrators, the "right" way was to keep control of women's bodies *out* of the state's hands.

Debates over authority in the field of reproductive health in Mexico are often tied to questions of authenticity: what is the authentic way to practice midwifery, to teach it, or even to write about it as an anthropologist? Despite recognizing that authenticity itself is a limited and potentially harmful descriptor because of its assumptions about the static or "pure" nature of knowledge and practice (assumptions which do not take into account the ways that knowledge and practice are not bound by geography or limited by time), I address these questions here because of their centrality to debates among midwives and scholars.

First, can students who do not entirely reflect the backgrounds of their patients still provide appropriate, quality care? I argue that they can and must: until there are better opportunities for education among marginalized communities in Mexico, professional training that comes with a living wage remains elusive for many. Some of the midwifery students did come from relatively privileged backgrounds, yet they entered into a profession whose rewards were sold to them in terms of helping others, not financial gain. Second, can NGOs whose leaders and funding sources do not entirely emerge from the communities where they work offer meaningful services? The rest of this book makes the case that they can; each of the schools described brings something important to the conversation about women's health care in Mexico and beyond. With their foreign influences they bring foreign ideas for treatment as well, but such has been the history of medicine: remedies and techniques travel and have always traveled. Of course, we should continue to pay attention to attempts to import ideas about health, bodies, education, and care and to hold individuals, NGOs, and the state accountable for addressing what actual women need and want.

As an anthropologist I make no claims to authenticity; my perspective is necessarily partial and situated (Haraway 1988), informed by my own experiences and positionality, though both have been shaped by my nearly twenty years spent working with midwives in Mexico. I have tried here to contextualize what I learned during that time within broader sociopolitical contexts but also to bring awareness to the daily challenges and accomplishments—big and small—playing out in homes, clinics, and midwifery schools.

Organization of the Book

The chapters that follow draw heavily from ethnographic data to show how midwives work both with and against the health-care system. These chapters highlight midwives' critiques of the very system they are trying to remain a part of—from its infrastructural failings that leave Indigenous women birthing outside on hospital lawns, to its entrenched obstetric violence against poor, rural women, to its lack of attention to gynecological health beyond the moment of procreation. They also show how midwives and midwifery schools are addressing these critiques through varied approaches that draw on both local and global knowledge.

Chapter 1, "Midwifery in Mexico and Beyond," begins with a question: what does midwifery even mean—historically, as well as in today's rapidly changing, globalizing, and increasingly biomedical context? In this chapter, we listen in as CASA's founder, Nadine, tries to answer this question for a group of incoming midwifery students. Her central premise is that midwifery is and has always been a profession that addresses social justice concerns. In examining what she means, I trace the history of midwives in Mexico and their complicated interactions with national and global health policies. I show how midwifery today is a product of these interactions, and those who study midwifery in Mexico today do so in response to the health and social justice needs they see in their communities as having been equally shaped by such policies.

In Chapter 2, "Breaking out of the 'Uterus Box,'" I show how global health policies that have prioritized maternal mortality reduction as the primary indicator of women's health have left many women's needs and desires behind. The title of the chapter references one school administrator's assertion that development policies focusing on birth to the exclusion of other health issues have kept women in the "uterus box." A global health and development emphasis on maternal mortality reduction has brought necessary attention to issues around pregnancy and birth, but the midwives argue that women's entire reproductive lives (not just their pregnancies and births) must be improved if real change is to happen. I describe how the Mujeres Aliadas school is trying to expand midwives' scope of practice to encompass holistic gynecological care. After witnessing women falling through the cracks in the health-care system, midwives there have taken matters into their own hands to conduct lab tests and get women quality care.

Chapters 3 and 4 reveal systemic forms of violence that permeate women's experiences of care in Mexico and show how midwives there are pushing back against them. Chapter 3, "Maternal Conditions," examines the ways that infrastructure changes meant to improve women's health outcomes (largely related to shifting birth from the home to the hospital) have also created conditions within which women are unable to receive the best care. Here, I tell the story of Irma, an Indigenous woman who was told to travel a great distance to give birth in a state hospital, only to be turned away and ultimately give birth outside on the patio. Like many Mexican women, Irma was told that the safest place to birth would be at the state hospital, not in her village with her local midwife. She did everything that was asked of her, yet her outcome was still dramatic and inhumane. I then describe the ways that midwives attempt to fill in the gaps that infrastructural failings have made, and I discuss how these failings must be understood as examples of "infrastructural violence." Infrastructural violence refers to the build environment (such as roads, clinics, or radio towers) and systems (such as the health-care system or the education system) that make structural violence against marginalized populations possible and, sometimes, inevitable. Chapter 4, "Obstetrics in a Time of Violence," focuses on the ways that gender violence—in the form of what midwives call *violencia obstétrica* (obstetric violence)—has become tied to biomedical interventions and institutions meant to improve women's health. Through the eyes of the midwifery students who work in public hospitals during their training at the CASA school of professional midwifery, I show how this obstetric violence reflects broader gendered, racial, and class inequalities in Mexico. Further, I show how midwifery students are confronting the effects of patterns of social violence and discrimination on women's bodies while working within the very systems where these most jarring patterns emerge.

In Chapter 5, "Modern Tradition," I look at traditional midwives and traditional midwifery practices that persist in Mexico today and argue that, rather than standing in as stoic relics of an ancient past, these practices persist because they respond to modern problems, often brought on by the work of development initiatives, and because they treat modern bodies whose conditions have been made possible in part because of the kinds of infrastructures, attitudes, and policies described in the previous chapters. This chapter centers on a traditional midwifery conference in Chiapas and highlights the simultaneous rootedness and globalness of the knowledge and practices shared by conference attendees. It also examines the model of the Nueve Lunas midwifery school in Oaxaca City, Oaxaca, as an approach that tries to bridge local needs with global knowledge.

In the Conclusion, "Creating Demand and Demanding Change," I recognize that despite the continued relevance of midwifery in Mexico and globally, midwives need to continuously reaffirm their worth. Part of this work involves the need to convince policy makers—as well as women and communities—that midwifery is a viable, safe option that can offer them a high quality of care while promising measurably better outcomes. I describe a theater production done at CASA that presented this message creatively, alongside official talks given by prominent politicians, promising to invest in midwifery's future. For midwifery to achieve its goals of improved quality of care and better health outcomes, midwives will need support from all levels. To gain this support, they need visibility.

The midwives I describe at the beginning of this Introduction, Juana and Elena, were quietly practicing their craft in the small village where they had lived all their lives. Yet each of them was in consistent contact with those who wanted to teach them and with those who wanted to learn from them (like me). Not all midwives seek out official state support or attend formal schools to get degrees and a state salary, yet those who do not find it increasingly difficult to continue to practice. This book is not the story of those midwives; though it includes some of their voices, I recognize that my research has focused primarily on the experiences of midwives associated with midwifery schools. While I started this research with intentions to trace the ways midwives learn across Mexico, I kept coming back to the schools. It was within those schools—written into the curricula, played out in the classrooms, debated among education and health officials—that I saw the swirling together of traditional practices, local necessities, and global aspirations.

The status of midwifery education in Mexico is changing rapidly, as schools try out new curricula and various states have begun opening their own professional midwifery training programs. However, this book presents a snapshot of how three very different midwifery schools emerged to address Mexico's legacy of inequality, gender violence, and health disparity. With this book I move beyond debates over educational standards and certification requirements (which certainly matter and which the individual schools and educators I worked with continue to revisit) and instead argue that midwifery writ large continues to exist and persist because it emphasizes the value of all women's needs and experiences.

Midwifery in Mexico and Beyond

What even is a midwife? This is a question that I heard answered in many different ways by many types of people over the years I spent in Mexico. In English, the term "midwife" derives from the expression for "with woman," and thus conveys a companion, someone who is (literally and figuratively) on the patient's side. In French, the term is *sage-femme*, or "wise woman," which defines her in terms of her knowledge. In Spanish, a midwife is a *partera*. Literally, this means a birth person, or a person who does births, though sometimes she is referred to as a *compañera* (companion), *comadrona*, or *comadre* (close friend). When the students I observed signed up to go to school to become midwives in Mexico, they had some notion of what the word meant but did not necessarily share the same vision for what their job would actually entail. Further, the definitions the students held for midwifery did not always align with (or, at least, start out aligned with) those held by their teachers and school administrators. It was through their educational journeys that many students became oriented toward a vision of midwifery that was about more than just delivering babies. Over the years that I spent observing with midwifery students of varied backgrounds across Mexico, I watched as they went from viewing a midwife as someone who was with women in the moment of birth to someone who was with women in a much broader sense—as an ally for women's rights both during and beyond reproduction.

In this chapter, I take as a starting point the notion that midwifery—no matter which set of techniques it uses, which types of licensure it seeks—is unique among medical professions because it is tied to issues of social justice. The midwife, because of the patients she tends to and her own historically marginalized professional position, has her work cut out for her: not only does she need to maintain her practice, but she also has to constantly do the work of fighting for her patients and her profession in a system that is frequently stacked against them both (Dixon, El Kotni, and Miranda 2019). In studying how midwives learn to be midwives, I was also studying how they learn what a midwife even is and why she matters. The varied educational programs being developed by the schools that I studied each oriented their students in different ways toward these questions, even as they navigated a balance between responding to national and global objectives on the one hand and the needs of their communities (which were not always fully valued by those objectives) on the other. Their divergence in approaches mirrors that found on a global scale: how midwives are trained, what they need to know, and how they are ultimately allowed to practice are all issues that reflect diverse social conditions.

Medical anthropologists have long been interested in how medical practitioners learn to be medical practitioners and in what happens during their transition from layperson to professional (Davis-Floyd 1987; Good and Del Vecchio Good 1993; Smith-Oka and Marshalla 2019). I watched as the midwifery students learned to see not only the human body differently through their training but also what their profession meant to their patients and communities. As I witnessed these transitions, I began to think about all of the ways that the design of the schools—from their curricula to their physical structures—reinforced the vision that midwifery students were learning what midwives should know, how they should practice, and what their larger purpose was. Of course, some days they were just learning to suture or read a lab test: the simplicity of a learnable skill. But other days were steeped in work with a different level of significance, as students were tasked with helping patients who were more in need of housing or a roof than prenatal vitamins, or when students interacted with hospital personnel who treated them (and their patients) poorly because of their race or gender. I watched as students learned through all of these educational moments—formal and informal—and saw as they began to build a vision of their profession that was woven through with awareness of social inequalities. But this awareness came later for most students. Even for those who came to midwifery explicitly because of a desire to help those without access to care in their communities, there were lessons to learn about the broader context of health, education, and inequality in Mexico.

"Part of a Movement Now": Midwifery as a Social Justice Movement

I was excited to meet the new cohort of students at the CASA midwifery school in San Miguel de Allende, where I had been working and doing research for some time, as it was always interesting to hear from them what they imagined midwifery to be all about when they first began their program of study. As described in the Introduction, CASA required relatively little of its incoming students: they were supposed to be eighteen, have completed middle school, have some passion for women's health, and (ideally) have a family connection to midwifery. I had met a variety of young women over the years who ended up at midwifery school who fit CASA's profile to varying degrees—seventeen year olds squeaking in under the age requirement because they really wanted to get out of their small towns; middle-aged women with master's degrees from Mexico City who had experienced natural birth and fallen in love with the idea of it; women who had wanted to be doctors or nurses but didn't finish high school or get good enough grades. The early weeks with a new cohort were interesting, watching such a range of students find common ground. When I heard that CASA's co-founder, Nadine, was going to speak to the new students, to give them her speech about what it meant to be a midwife, I knew I wanted to attend.

It was a long, hot walk from downtown San Miguel de Allende up the hill to the CASA midwifery school that sat perched on the city's hilly outskirts. The startlingly cool air and burst of chattering voices echoing against cement walls hit me simultaneously as I slipped into the classroom. Students from each year of the program already filled the brightly painted wooden chairs that surrounded the central table serving as their communal desk, and many more students lined the edges of the room. I found a sliver of floor space and settled in amid my bags, notebooks, and layers of clothing, greeting and smiling at the students around me. I had observed enough classes to know that the arrival of the teacher did not usually lead to a silencing of the group, but today—despite the number of students packed into the room—an expectant quiet descended when Nadine walked in.

Nadine did not often address the students during classroom time. She was not a midwife herself, so she left most teaching to the medical professionals. Trained in public health and social work and from New York City, she had lived and worked in Mexico for more than thirty years and had seen CASA grow from its modest beginnings into an established NGO with international donors and write-ups in the *New York Times*. Today's meeting had been planned for Nadine to give the students an overview of the history of midwifery in Mexico, the history of CASA, and the school's goals for the future. After opening with some casual introductions and checking in with the new students about how they were feeling about the year so far (they were only a couple of months into the semester), she jumped right in to the main point of her talk.

"The key word here is *movimiento* (movement)," she exclaimed, pausing to let the word sink in. "You are all a part of a movement now. I hope you know that you are not here as students, but as activists. If you don't know that yet, then we at the school have not done our jobs." The students smiled at this, but looked slightly confused. They had indeed not been told that they were here as activists, at least not the new students who had not heard Nadine talk before. That was not part of the regular recruitment rhetoric. I could see some of the younger and more shy students look uneasily at each other. Seventeen- or eighteen-year-old young women straight off the ranch from Chiapas or Veracruz had not signed on as activists but rather as novice midwives. They had imagined patient care, not picket lines.

"This job is not *just* about loving and caring for women," Nadine continued. "You have to know what is going on in Mexico and in the world. You need to know the history of this profession. You have to understand the situation around maternal mortality, around education, around poverty in Mexico. But more than just knowing about these topics in general, you have to know the *numbers*. You cannot be respected if you do not know the numbers." From there, Nadine turned on her laptop and began a lengthy slide presentation that brought the numbers to life. I watched as students scrambled to pull notebooks out of bags and begin to take notes. They were being given a lecture on why midwifery matters but also a lesson on how to convey midwifery's significance to those who care less about "loving and caring for women" than they do about the statistics.

In the next section, I examine how Mexico's relationship to midwifery has shifted over time in response to global pressures, then describe the different approaches to midwifery training that inform this book. By situating these educational options within the shifting global recommendations for midwives, I show how Mexican midwives are strategically working both with and against these shifts as they define what they think midwives should know, how they should learn, and where they should practice. In doing the work of defining modern midwifery, they take on the mantle of activism within a framework of reproductive justice, whether they want to or not; the health of their patients and the future of their profession depend on their ability to advocate for better options in women's health care and to demonstrate that hiring midwives makes the most sense as a way to provide those options in Mexico today.

"Midwives Have Always Existed": The Dynamic but Consistent Presence of Midwifery in Mexico

The role of midwifery has changed in many ways over Mexico's history, especially in terms of the relationships midwives have had with the Mexican government and formal health-care system. When Nadine's students seemed surprised at her declaration that midwifery is first and foremost a social movement, they revealed that their understanding of what midwives are and do reflects only one way that midwives have been seen in Mexico. They had come to CASA to learn to be "professional midwives," a career that many of them told me they saw leading to stable jobs in health centers. Many others told me that they planned to return to their communities, in Veracruz or Chiapas or Oaxaca, and set up their own private practice. What the majority of new midwifery students did not realize was that by even choosing to become a "professional" midwife (that is, with a recognized degree instead of an inherited title), they were already stepping into the political spotlight. As Nadine would remind them, Mexico had its eyes on them from the start. That is in part because of the different roles midwives have played historically and in part because of the hopes that people like Nadine had for the roles midwives could play going forward.

Within current Mexican midwifery circles, there is frequent debate over the terms used for practitioners. Calling oneself (or another midwife) "traditional" (*partera tradicional* or *comadrona*), "professional" (*partera profesional*), or "empirical" (*partera empírica*) can mean very different things to different people.[1] Indeed, after a heated debate one afternoon between one group of midwives discussing whether they should be able to call themselves "professional midwives" if they did not have a government title to that effect, one midwife threw up her hands and asked, rhetorically, "Why can't we just be midwives without last names (*parteras sin apellidos*)?" Her exasperated request reflected the hierarchical tensions that the various names could instill, even among groups of similarly minded midwives. Throughout this book, I use the terms "professional midwife" and "traditional midwife" when they were meaningfully employed by the midwives themselves to connote what they saw as an important distinction in their training or job scope. However, I also use the term "midwife" (without a last name), because the midwives in this book saw themselves as having a shared identity as midwives (*parteras*) that bridged professional/traditional divides, and in regular conversation they referred to themselves as such.

Confusion over what to call midwives extends beyond Mexico. This confusion stems from historically shifting definitions of who should attend births, what they need to know, and where they should work. In her talk with the CASA students, Nadine framed the current state of midwifery in Mexico within a broader historical trajectory: "We must always remember," she told them, "that midwives have always existed, as long as humans have." The history of Mexican midwifery has long been interconnected with the changing roles midwives have played globally.

Midwifery was a long-standing recognized profession in Mexico before the Spanish arrived. In pre-Hispanic times, midwives worked not only with women in birth, but also as community and religious leaders and as health educators and priestesses (Castañeda Núñez 1988). During the colonial period, midwifery continued as a respected profession. Indigenous, Spanish, black, *mestizo*, and *mulata* midwives practiced their trade for centuries, even after Mexico's independence from Spain. Mexican scholar Ana María Carrillo (1999) has written one of the only comprehensive accounts of the history of midwives after the arrival of the Spanish. During early colonization in Mexico, women sought out the care of midwives based on their experience in everything from childbirth to fertility concerns, milk production, miscarriages, and postpartum support. In 1750, Spain ordered that all its colonies would require midwives to be certified—a process which required them to have studied for four years with an approved teacher, show their marriage license or prove their status as a widow, prove that they had been baptized, and pay a fee (León 1910, 227).

As Nadine took the students through this history, she emphasized to them that the idea of "professionalizing" midwives is not new; while their own school, CASA, was still fighting for legitimacy and recognition, she wanted them to know that the idea of professionally trained midwives had roots in Mexico. "In 1833," she told them, "the first medical school created the idea of professional midwifery training, and in 1841 the first student got her title there. Between 1841 and 1888, 140 midwives went through that program!" For Nadine, this was proof that, at least for a time, there was support for such training for midwives. Midwifery was supported as a career for women in Mexico because it reflected the appropriate virtues women were seen to hold.

In a history of medicine in Mexico from 1886, author Francisco A. Flores elaborated on what he saw as this natural rationale for women to refrain from most of the medical professions of the time:

> Because imagination and feeling dominate in the weaker sex, perhaps in the theoretical studies of medicine women could be distinguished; but in practice, in this tremendous practice that sometimes puts in the doctor's hand the homicidal knife and urges him to act without delay; in that practice that sometimes demands such cold blood and such serenity, that even man may lack, and a decision and an indifference to suffering, that women do not have nor could have, and it would be an absurdity to require it of her. (264; my translation)

Flores went on to note that women should dedicate themselves instead to music, painting, or literature, which he argued were more in line with their nature. Among women, however, Flores noted an important distinction: "If we say this about women in general, we especially refer to the Latin race, the most intelligent but the most sensitive" (265; my translation). In addition to the arts, however, Flores did note that midwifery was an appropriate vocation for women, and it was seen as quite distinct from other more specialized fields of medicine, such as those that could involve surgery.

One interesting problem for early midwifery training was that there were few maternity hospitals, except in larger cities with established midwifery training programs. In order to be licensed, midwives had to get a year of practical experience either under a physician or an approved midwife, which proved difficult initially, as their schools were purely theory based. It was not until the mid-1800s that maternity hospitals became common across Mexico, usually associated with medical schools, where midwives and doctors alike were able to conduct their clinical observations. Many women patients complained about the treatment they received from students and doctors there, but the trend was already set in motion to move birth into hospital centers and out of the home (Carrillo 1999). Nadine put it more forcefully during an interview, arguing that "putting licensed midwives in the hospitals was part of the public health system's plan. Women didn't trust hospitals in those days, but they trusted the midwives, and so they went, which was how the hospital became a normal place to go for birth.

The midwives were used, they were like '*un gancho que hizo que la gente se acostumbrara a ir al hospital*' (a hook that made people get used to going to the hospital)!"

Midwives did not work to "hook" women into going to hospitals solely based on their imagined distinction from biomedical practitioners, however. Rather than simply distrusting doctors in favor of their local midwives for epistemological ideas, women were reacting to complex historical legacies: for decades, efforts to bring medical teams into rural areas "arrived as one element in a raft of state assumptions over socio-economic hierarchy, land tenure, and political obedience. As a result, the diffusion of rural health care closely paralleled the penetration of the Mexican state, creating inequalities in access to health care in different areas," such that for those areas that had complied with state rules, health care was better than in regions where people had resisted (in which case medical teams could take decades to return) (Smith 2012, 41).

I think it is worth pausing to think about the image of the hook and how it has been used to visualize the work that midwives have long done for the Mexican state. Midwives were seen as *un gancho*, a hook that pulled women out of their rural lives and into the state clinics and hospitals for birth. Yet this was not the idea of the midwives themselves; they were not moving to hospital-based practice in the hopes of luring their patients there and then stepping aside in a bait-and-switch move that would only benefit the doctors. Midwives have had many reasons to want to work in hospitals—from professional legitimacy to employment security to financial reasons to patient desires—but it would not have made sense for them to knowingly participate in a project of self-erasure. Further, this project never fully succeeded; despite being used as hooks to some extent to get women to birth with doctors instead of midwives, midwifery persists both inside and outside hospital settings. A hook can bring someone in, but it can also hold them—perhaps midwives have also been able to maintain a hold on women to some degree. I think that throughout the decades when women were being pushed into hospital births, midwives continued to offer alternative types of treatment, local options for care, and a humanized approach to birth that appealed to many women and sometimes was the only option.

Still, state efforts largely succeeded in normalizing hospital births and disseminating messages that discredited midwives as legitimate professionals. Many midwives had attended the state-supported schools but had never received an official title, and they were the first to be critiqued as illegitimate. However, once the specialty of gynecology was born in medical schools in 1887, even the licensed midwives were discredited. In 1892, the federal government published its intent to officially replace licensed midwives with doctors but continue to use the midwives to "convince patients and their families of the importance of using medical services" (Carrillo 1999, 178; my translation). With this shift, midwives' scope of practice was restricted to only low-risk births. They had to refer any possible complications to the doctors who now supervised their practices (Carrillo 1999). In the late 1800s, midwives appealed to the state to recognize that they indeed had better training and outcomes than medical students and that they should be allowed to attend births as they had been trained to do, yet their request was denied by the secretary of justice under Porfirio Díaz (Penyak 2003, 66). "You have to remember," Nadine told her students at CASA, "that by 1900 there were almost as many midwives in Mexico as doctors." As such, this refusal to allow them to do the work they had trained to do was doubly demeaning; they were not a small fringe group of practitioners with a long history of serving women and communities. The way that the state systematically cut them out of their profession continues to haunt the current moment of tenuous new ties between Mexican midwives and the state.

For a time during the late 1800s, programs continued to exist that produced licensed midwives, but the subject matter that students had to learn became increasingly esoteric—including, for example, such seemingly tangential requirements as two years of French lessons (France was heavily idolized by President Porfirio Díaz, who saw all things French as indications of modernity, despite having never been there until his own exile in 1911) (Priego 2008). The political battle continued, with physicians pushing the state to designate them as certified primary providers for pregnancy and birth (Carrillo 1999). This was at a time when doctors held great political sway. The School of Medicine was a central locus of power under Díaz, and politicians and scientists (including doctors) enjoyed a mutually beneficial relationship in which scientists lent credibility to politicians' modernization initiatives in exchange for funding from the state (Priego 2008).[2] It was no surprise, then, that doctors successfully achieved the designation as reproductive care providers, after which point they began charging very high prices for their services, beyond what most poor women could afford (Carrillo 1999). The doctors argued that their approach was safer and more scientific (a concept Díaz strongly supported) (Priego 2008) and that the midwives' use of techniques such as plants, vertical birth positions, shawls, and external rotations of the fetus were dangerous, old fashioned, ignorant, and vulgar (Carrillo 1999; Flores 1886).[3] Doctors needed to distinguish themselves from this vision of midwifery, to prove that their methods were more modern. When things went wrong in births attended by midwives, physicians characterized them as ignorant; when things went wrong for the doctors, they blamed it on "a force of nature or the limitations of science" (Carrillo 1999, 186). It is worth noting that general practice doctors in Mexico are granted the official degree of a Licenciatura en Médico, Cirujano y Partero (Bachelor's Degree in Medicine, Surgery, and Midwifery). That midwifery became officially tied to the medical degree reflects the institutionalized attempt to shift birth to the physician's realm.

Despite the politics, there remained roughly the same number of licensed midwives as doctors in Mexico at the beginning of the twentieth century. But things began to change rapidly as the century progressed, in conjunction with other political and social shifts as Mexico transitioned out of Porfirio Díaz's reign and into the Mexican Revolution (1910–1917). The social Darwinism promoted by Díaz's *científicos* had led to decades of neglect of large swaths of the population, under the belief that the poor and Indigenous were "destined to die out" (Coerver, Pasztor, and Buffington 2004, 141). Where Díaz had viewed science, modernity, and education as belonging to the urban elite, the revolution and subsequent presidents called for access to such engines of progress for all Mexicans, including the rural poor (Priego 2008). A growing national emphasis on public health, framed largely in terms of hygiene awareness, emerged during the revolution and promised to finally carry Mexico into modernity in a way that Díaz's more elitist views of science had not (Aréchiga Córdoba 2005).[4] While much of the post-revolution campaigns focused on bringing health and hygiene to Mexico's rural poor as a way of modernizing the country as a whole, the 1916 book *La higiene en México* (Hygiene in Mexico) by Alberto J. Pani argued that it was in part due to Díaz's corruption that even Mexico's great cities boasted mortality rates two to three times higher than cities in the United States or Europe (Aréchiga Córdoba 2005). One way to remedy this, and to thus bring Mexico in line with the modern world, was through health and hygiene propaganda campaigns and the expansion of public health services. Within this vision, midwives occupied a questionable position: they provided important health services, but they did not necessarily fit the image of modernity that the state was going for. A 1928 propaganda campaign by the secretary of public education, for example, targeted the Indigenous population specifically in telling them not to use traditional practices, such as putting urine or feces on wounds, using herbal remedies, or making potions (Aréchiga Córdoba 2005, 140); while such a depiction made a caricature of traditional healing practices, it also made clear that practitioners (like midwives) who used them were not in line with the modern health and hygiene campaigns.

In the 1930s, building on ideas about the need to modernize Mexico beyond its urban centers through more involved health care and health education, a plan was devised to establish more than one hundred rural health centers (Soto Laveaga 2013). Through this expansion of state health care into rural communities, of which prenatal and birth care was a part, some communities were slowly introduced to the idea that modern citizens seek maternal health care at state clinics—not with traditional village midwives. Over the following decades, even midwives practicing in urban hospitals faced increasing limitations on the medical procedures they could perform, and hospitals stopped hiring them. After 1960, any midwives still working in hospitals were no longer allowed to attend births (Carrillo 1999).

Throughout this process of exclusion, traditional midwives continued to attend the majority of births outside hospitals. In 1911, following the opening of the first national nursing schools, midwives were told that they must have a nursing degree in order to be licensed (Carrillo 1999, 188), but the reality was that most midwives continued to work for decades in regions where such training was not possible, even if they would have wanted to do it. Whole swaths of the country did not even have access to doctors or hospitals for most of the twentieth century (indeed, access to care continues to be an important factor across Mexico); in 1951 there was only one hospital in the state of Chiapas, and the state of Veracruz still had twenty times the number of state clinics that states like Guerrero, Oaxaca, or Campeche had in 1965 (Smith 2012, 41).[5] Even in regions where there were hospitals or clinics, not everyone could afford to go there. It was not until 1943, when the Ministry of Health created the Mexican Social Security Institute (IMSS), that private-sector workers and their families had insurance, and not until 1959 that the Institute of Social Services and Security for Civil Servants (ISSSTE) was created for government employees and their families to get health care (Knaul and Frenk 2005).[6] These programs dovetailed with a growing global emphasis on national health outcomes as measures of development, through such organizations as the United Nations (founded in 1945) (Baker Opperman 2012). Social insurance did not arrive across Mexico all at once, however, with implementation concentrating initially in urban regions; indeed, in Oaxaca, for example, IMSS was not available until 1952 (Dion 2008; Fajardo-Ortiz 2008).

With the arrival of IMSS to rural Mexico, the idea that prenatal care and childbirth should take place in the clinic, rather than with a community midwife, was just one of many ideas about hygiene, illness prevention, and social norms that practitioners promoted. However, even into the 1980s, more than half of births in Mexico took place outside hospitals (COPLA-MAR 1983). Brigitte Jordan argued in her 1978 seminal book, *Birth in Four Cultures*, that traditional midwives persisted in Mexico because they offered culturally appropriate support for women, even if they did not have the same technical medical training. They also persisted in such numbers at that time because, given the slow and uneven pace of biomedical expansion, they were still called on by women who had no other options or had yet to be convinced otherwise.

The story of why women began going in greater numbers to clinics and hospitals to give birth (rather than doing it at home) is thus in part related to this expansion of the biomedical presence across Mexico. It is also, however, part of a bigger shift in public perceptions around hospitals that had begun in the nineteenth and early twentieth centuries in Mexico and beyond.[7] With the advent of "new midwifery" training coming out of Europe in the early nineteenth century, physicians began to advertise techniques and technologies (such as forceps for addressing difficult deliveries and ether and chloroform for pain reduction) that addressed the very real concerns women had about complications and pain in labor (Thomasson and Treber 2008). As medical training began focusing increasingly on clinical experience, doctors began pushing women to be seen at the hospital rather than at home; for doctors, it began to seem easier and possibly more lucrative to attend to patients at fixed locations with nursing staff, modern medical technologies, and beds that made for easier forceps access (Risse 1999; Thomasson and Treber 2008). For women, the idea had spread by the early twentieth century that it was safer to deliver in hospitals than at home because of the technologies doctors offered there, despite the finding that such deliveries did not necessarily improve women's health outcomes at that time (Hausman 2005, Thomasson and Treber 2008, Walzer Leavitt 2016).

As the perceptions of hospitals shifted from places for the destitute to places that provided the latest in medical technologies and offered safer outcomes, hospital births became increasingly normalized. In the United

States this shift was quite rapid: between 1900 and 1935, the percentage of hospital births in the United States rose from 5 percent to 50 percent (and 75 percent in urban regions) (Thomasson and Treber 2008, 77). In Mexico, this same trend led to a steady decline in home births attended by midwives throughout the twentieth century. By the mid-1990s traditional midwives attended less than 17 percent of Mexican births (Davis-Floyd 2001a). In 2014, this number had dropped even more: 94.6 births were attended by doctors, and only 2.7 were attended by a traditional or professional midwife (Senado de la República 2017). The continuing pressure on women to seek out biomedical care for their births or risk being labeled as noncompliant or disobedient reflects the way that state projects intersect with women's choices and ultimately shape their health experiences and outcomes (Smith-Oka 2012).

As scholars have pointed out, across Latin America—and, indeed, across the world—when midwives are pushed out of regular practice, they are left to attend only the most life-endangering of births, those that occur in emergency situations, such as twins or a breech baby, or when the patient cannot get to a doctor (Davis-Floyd et al. 2009, 11). This is in direct conflict with the agenda supported by many politicians today to have midwives attending only low-risk births, if any. Yet in Mexico's marginalized communities, women can suddenly find themselves in labor and in trouble if they cannot get to a clinic in time for a number of reasons, including bad roads, lack of transportation, or simply a lack of time. This is concerning because it means that midwives are not regularly attending births, yet their quick thinking and skills are being called on in much more serious cases.

Mexico's decline in traditional midwives is exacerbated by the aging of midwives and the lack of apprentices to whom they may pass their knowledge. Further affecting midwifery's decline are Mexican trends in formal education and attitudes about the progressive nature of hospitals over what are seen as alternative healing practices. People don't always want to go to midwives anymore, especially when state health-care services are free and they are told that midwives are dangerous.

Another factor that lead to the decline in the kind of midwifery that was long practiced in Mexico was the *capacitaciones* (trainings). These short-term, government-led training modules for rural and traditional midwives began to take the place of the more formalized licensure programs during the first half of the twentieth century (El Kotni 2019). These programs continue today, often as periodic, short training modules (Davis-Floyd 2001a), and academics studying these trainings around the world as well as the midwives I worked with have been quick to criticize them as ineffective and, in some cases, dangerous (El Kotni 2016, 2018). Stacy Pigg, for example, has written about attempts to export biomedical training to traditional workers in Nepal. The result of such programs, she finds, is that the Indigenous people learn to talk like their trainers want them to in order to pass as participants in the biomedical model, as legitimate care providers, even if their practices continue to diverge from the training standards. Therefore, despite the trend in international health programs to appreciate other types of knowledge, the "training programs continue to serve the 'cosmopolitical' function of establishing medical obstetrics as authoritative" (1997, 234).

The idea of the traditional birth attendant (TBA) as a practitioner who received some form of these less official trainings took hold on a global scale in the 1970s and 1980s as a way to quickly train lay health providers in the hopes of improving maternal health. The World Health Organization supported the idea of TBA trainings in developing regions worldwide on how to deal with obstetric emergencies, detect complications, treat infections and hemorrhages, and perform other potentially life-saving techniques (Lane and Garrod 2016). At the International Safe Motherhood Initiative Conference in 1987 (which was sponsored by such global partners as the World Bank, the WHO, the International Planned Parenthood Federation, the Population Council, and UNFPA), a clear global goal was set for reducing maternal mortality by half by the year 2000. The route to achieving this goal was determined: training TBAs was to be a priority (Summer, Walker, and Guendelman 2019, 64–65). This landmark global decision to back TBAs shaped the trainings for midwives for many years to follow. Yet the way these trainings proceeded was never standardized.

Fernanda, a professional midwife herself and then director of CASA, told me in 2009 that traditional midwives—who were considered the TBAs—in Mexico have been irrevocably harmed because of such trainings. "Since 1972," she said, "the government began rounding up midwives and giving them brief workshops. They would just tell them things like 'external rotations are dangerous,' or 'just use oxytocin.'" For Fernanda, these trainings were both the wrong kind of information and the wrong method of training—by only telling the traditional midwives to do certain things but not giving them the background or tools to understand when and why to do them, they were destroying many of the practices and much of the knowledge passed down over centuries that were connected to the needs and resources within their communities.

TBAs and SBAs: Shifting Priorities for Midwifery Training on the Global Level

It did not take long for global health organizations to reverse their posi-tion on the training of TBAs. Just a few years after the International Safe Motherhood Initiative Conference that had called on countries to invest in TBA training as a way to improve maternal health outcomes, the gravity of the global maternal mortality crisis was revealed by the WHO in 1990, and TBAs' lack of systematic training or scientific knowledge was largely blamed (Summer, Walker, and Guendelman 2019, 65). Suddenly, TBAs went from being heralded as local champions of women's health to being explic-itly rebranded as unskilled and potentially dangerous. In Mexico, this shift aligned with the government push to get women away from midwives and into state clinics and hospitals for births and gave fuel to the public health workers who were tasked with visiting pregnant women and telling them not to deliver with their local midwife. Over and over again, during my years working with and visiting midwives around Mexico, I would hear them recount how their patients had been told not to see them anymore, that the midwives were not only unskilled, but that they might kill their babies.

Skilled birth attendants (SBAs) became the new game in town. When the United Nations developed its Millennium Development Goal to reduce maternal mortality by 75 percent between 2000 and 2015, TBAs were explic-itly not counted as SBAs (Summer, Walker, and Guendelman 2019, 67). In 2004, the WHO, along with the International Confederation of Midwives (ICM) and the International Federation of Gynecology and Obstetrics (FIGO) set forth the definition of an SBA as: "A midwife, doctor, or nurse—who has been educated and trained to proficiency in the skills needed to man-age normal (uncomplicated) pregnancies, childbirth, and the immediate postnatal period, and in the identification, management, and referral of complications in women and newborns" (WHO 2004, 1; quoted in Hobbs et al. 2019, 2).

TBAs, the report said, had not been shown to reduce maternal deaths. Indeed, the report urged countries to avoid the "trap" of trying to train TBAs to deal with maternal health issues—doing so would result in a waste of resources that should instead be dedicated to establishing formal training programs for SBAs. TBAs could continue to work in women's health, but their role should be "as an advocate for skilled care, encouraging women to seek care from skilled attendants" (WHO 2004, 8). The midwifery schools described in this book, despite having diverse curricula, all provided the kind of formalized training that seemed to align with the global push for SBAs. The fact that they all approached training so differently reflects what has been found on a global scale, as well; how SBAs are named, trained, and allowed to practice varies widely (Hobbs et al. 2019).

More recent studies, however, have shown that this global plan to divert energy away from TBAs and toward SBAs has had uneven results, which stem from two important sources: on the one hand, such efforts assumed a timeline for structural changes in educational and professional opportunities that was unrealistic,[8] and on the other hand, these efforts ignored the multifaceted and significant roles that TBAs play in their communities beyond care in pregnancy and birth (Lane and Garrod 2016). It seemed that the world was neither ready to do away with TBAs nor prepared to train and put to work a new generation of SBAs.

In light of these findings, countries are now being urged to reinvest in TBA trainings while slowly working toward the creation of sustainable SBA opportunities. This has been controversial—and, indeed, confusing, given the rapid about-face from prior anti-TBA sentiments—because TBAs had been cast as less skilled providers. Yet some argue that "better coverage in poor resource nations could be achieved by recognizing the skills of those already on the ground who, for many women, are currently the carer of choice for a variety of reasons" (Lane and Garrod 2016, 3). Indeed, a pilot study conducted in Guerrero, a state in southern Mexico, offered support, birthing space, and trained community health worker liaisons between TBAs and hospital services to a random selection of TBAs. They found that people accepted the intervention, women were not worse off, and there were significantly lower birth complications for the intervention communities. The authors attributed this improvement in complications to both the intercultural abilities of the community health workers and the increase in use of traditional midwives (Sarmiento et al. 2018). This study, though small, showed the potential for improved outcomes when TBAs were supported and connected to the health-care system.

An inherent difficulty in the discussions around TBAs and SBAs is that the semantic distinction pits "traditional" against "skilled." To be traditional, by this measure, is to be unskilled; on the other hand, to be skilled implies a distance from traditional methods. This same distinction arose frequently in the debates I heard among midwives over who should be called "professional midwives" and who should be called "traditional midwives" in Mexico, for again, to be traditional implies a lack of professionalism. For those who call midwifery their profession, this distinction can be demeaning. Further, the term "professional" means very different things to different midwives—for some, it means having attended an official educational program (like those described below), while for others it means having an explicitly biomedical training. This all gets further complicated when traditional midwives, like Juana (described in the Introduction), employ biomedical treatments like Pitocin because they went through the state-mandated TBA trainings.

Indeed, when looking back on Juana's liberal use of Pitocin, I can imagine her trajectory through such state workshops, in which the oxytocin-simulating drug was pushed on midwives as a wonder drug for laboring and postpartum women. Yet Pitocin is not a benign drug; indeed, when given incorrectly it can force the uterus to contract too strongly or for too prolonged a time, posing a threat to the mother and baby. On the one hand, Juana's participation in such workshops validated her practice and gave her authority within her community, yet on the other hand these workshops have been shown to provide a very uneven level of information and follow-through for their students, as well as uneven improvements in access to care for patients (El Kotni 2016, 2018; Miranda 2015). The outcome reflects a contradiction of modernization: the very practices, technologies, and beliefs attached to projects of national development in health often result in the devaluation of women's bodies and a decline in women's health outcomes and experiences.

Mexican midwives today are a product of these contradictions. While midwives stood for decades as examples of the antithesis of modernization, they are now being reconsidered as useful actors of development *because of* their ability to fill the gaps left by biomedical interventions. While this may seem counterintuitive, I think that—like the image of the hook—sometimes that which is meant to serve as one thing can become something else. The state set up midwives to stand for the antithesis of modernity, but now some state officials turn to midwives to address the very modern problems left in the wake of development policies. Midwives have thus reclaimed some measure of authority as agents of modernization, a claim that aligns them with a long-held national vision. This alignment challenges us to rethink modern midwifery as a profession that is savvy of evidence-based practices, speaks the language of global development, and offers a corrective to some of the negative impacts of decades of biomedical institutions and interventions. For the midwives in this book, how women experience birth matters to individual health outcomes, but it also holds the potential to enact social change. Rethinking midwives as modern practitioners challenges us to think about humane treatment of women in childbirth as itself a route to development.

Making Sense of Midwifery Education within the Mexican Educational Context

I was observing a class of third-year CASA students one afternoon when an unfamiliar woman entered the room. She was a visiting obstetrician, there to teach students some advanced materials in obstetrics. After plunking her stack of books down on the long wooden table that served as their communal desk, she scanned the room silently, imposing a layer of seriousness upon the students who, until she had arrived, had been happily chatting and laughing. As they fell silent, the teacher asked them, "You know this old saying: '*El bebé va a nacer con la partera, sin la partera, o a pesar de la partera,*' right?" The expression, which was sometimes tossed around derogatively, translates to, "the baby will be born with the midwife, without the midwife, or in spite of the midwife." It sends a clear message: midwives do not add anything to a birth and can sometimes get in the way. I had heard the expression in contexts where midwives' knowledge was in question—were they even learning the right things to do any good for women? The students that day in the classroom were immediately angered by the phrase, and this opening led the teacher to implore them to study hard and learn enough to dispel such beliefs about midwifery. "You have to know this information," she said, stabbing her obstetrics book with her index finger. That midwives had to know enough to improve women's health was clearly vital to their ability to practice and gain legitimacy in their field, but how they were to learn that was answered differently across the schools where I worked.

In addition to the work they do, the *way* midwives learn their profession is also part of a broader social movement. After years of observing the varied midwifery training programs around Mexico, I learned that school administrators, teachers, and students were all making important choices when it came to defining what midwives needed to know and how they should learn—choices that reflected their values, the needs of their communities, and the realities of the Mexican education system. In determining who gets to learn midwifery, what midwifery school should entail, and what career paths graduated midwives might follow, the schools I worked with had to figure out how to work with the health and education systems while simultaneously critiquing the lack of equality within these systems. If midwifery was to be accessible as a career path and create lasting social change, it would have to be offered in ways that did not simply recreate the divisions between rich and poor, rural and urban, or Indigenous and non-Indigenous found in Mexico's current education system.

In talking to midwifery students, I saw how their choice to study midwifery was inspired by many different factors, from family connections to the practice (which was what CASA had hoped for), to randomly encountering a brochure or website about the program. Many students, however, described their decision to study midwifery in terms of their inability to study other things because of the lack of educational opportunities in their communities.

"Why did you decide to study midwifery?" I asked a first-year student one afternoon, as she took a break from her studies on a bench outside a classroom at CASA, some months after Nadine's introductory talk. She looked over at her friend and giggled, then sort of shrugged and said to me, "Well, I wanted to study medicine, but there was no high school in my town. So, I didn't go to high school, and I didn't know what I was going to do. But then I saw something about CASA, so I came here." I nodded and asked, "So you wanted to be a doctor?" She replied yes, that had been her plan since she was young, to be a pediatrician, but she realized as she grew up how hard that would be. It became kind of a fantasy, she said—something that seemed impossible. Midwifery would not have occurred to her as something she could study, because she had not known that one could actually graduate with a real degree in midwifery and get paid a living salary. The opportunity she found at CASA would let her become a health-care practitioner, despite not having even a high-school diploma.

Not all of the midwifery schools allowed for students to enter without a high-school diploma, but CASA did—a fact that caused much debate among school administrators, politicians, and doctors, some of whom felt that a high-school education was a necessary prerequisite. However, one of the reasons that it continues to make sense to train midwives at various educational levels is that many people still do not have access to other forms of higher education that could lead, for example, to nursing or medical degrees. In this section I describe the education system in Mexico and show how the diverse midwifery training opportunities there fill a gap in educational and career opportunities, especially for young, rural women.

The education system is changing in Mexico, but change is slow to come to the country's most marginalized populations and regions. This should not come as a great surprise, given Mexico's historically unequal approach to public education. When, in 1883 under President Porfirio Díaz, a constitutional amendment was proposed that would make primary education mandatory for all Mexicans, public controversy over the value of educating the Indigenous people (who made up nearly half the population) sparked much debate (Powell 1968). It was not until 1888 that mandatory primary education was passed, though the roll out of this plan was slow and very uneven, especially for Indigenous Mexicans; indeed, many of the stifled pleas to Díaz to invest in education for Indigenous Mexicans would be taken up with more force during the Mexican Revolution after 1910 (Powell 1968).[9]

The Mexican education system is currently divided into primary school (grades one through six), secondary school (grades seven through nine), and high school (grades ten through twelve; depending on the type of program, this is referred to as *preparatoria*, *bachillerato*, or *educación media superior*). There is the option to pursue a technical, terminal degree (what is referred to in the United States as vocational school) for those who only finish secondary school. Students who then go on to college would earn an undergraduate degree (*licenciatura*), followed possibly by a masters (*maestría*) then doctorate (*doctorado*). Nursing programs vary (including degrees in *auxiliares de enfermería*, *técnicos en enfermería*, and *licenciaturas en enfermería*), and nurses may go on to get masters or doctoral degrees, as well. To become a medical doctor, students must pass a test to get into medical school after high school (without going to college first) then complete a year of internship and a year of social service. If they want to specialize, they must then compete for a residency in their desired specialization.

While the options for education appear well established, there are still many people who do not have access to education beyond primary or secondary school or who have to drop out in order to work. In 2016, more than half of young adults between twenty-five and thirty-four years old had not completed high school (OECD 2016). While this number has improved over the past decade, it is still quite high. The Mexican federal government announced in 2011 that states would have to start offering state-run high schools (they were previously only obligated to pay for education through middle school, making high school a cost that was put back onto families), but the reality of enacting this shift nationwide is daunting. Of those who did go on to higher education (beyond high school), in 2016, only 17 percent of adults between ages twenty-five and sixty-four had actually completed their degree (OECD 2016).

These numbers continue to lag for Indigenous populations in Mexico, and especially for Indigenous women. The majority of children classified as Indigenous in Mexico attend primary school, but after age fifteen their numbers drop off precipitously, such that in 2015, only 34 percent of the Indigenous population between ages fifteen and twenty-four was in school (compared to 44 percent of the general population in this age range at this time) (INPI 2018). Indigenous men are more likely to stay in school longer than Indigenous women, as well—a dynamic that is reflected in the finding that Indigenous Mexican women have an illiteracy rate of 22.2 percent, five points higher than that of Indigenous men (and much higher than the 5.5 percent illiteracy rate nationwide) (INPI 2018).

These differences in educational attainment map directly onto economic possibilities and contribute to the entrenched inequalities that carve deep divisions across Mexico and affect all aspects of life there. More education leads to significantly higher employment rates and higher pay: those who went to college earn double those who only completed high school, while those who have a masters or doctoral degree earn four times as much (OECD 2016). This means that those who have historically had less access to higher education (beyond middle school) are stuck in a cycle of not earning as much and not being able to offer their own children higher educational opportunities.

When Nadine framed midwifery as a social justice intervention, she was in part positioning it as a way to interrupt this cycle. Getting an education in midwifery would allow students to earn a living wage while also helping their communities through meaningful employment. Even for the other schools I studied that required a higher level of education to enter, the opportunity to get formal training that could lead to a stable job and give back to the community was framed as central to the educational project.

The diverse paths to midwifery education in Mexico reflected the uneven landscape of educational levels, opportunities, and access that would-be midwives had. One way that this diversity manifested was in differences regarding schools' relationships to formal state or national education systems. Some schools, like CASA, felt that the only way to really institutionalize midwifery as a valid career option and method of care in the state healthcare system, where most women went for health care already, was to formalize midwifery education through government licensure. An increasing number of schools based on CASA's model that have opened in the past decade hold a Registro de Validez Oficial de Estudios (RVOE). This means that graduates who complete their requirements are eligible to receive a federally recognized license (*cédula*) that allows them to practice in the public sector (Faget and Capasso 2017)—an option that many find appealing because it comes with a fixed salary (in 2011, this was set at 12,000 pesos a month, or about 960 US dollars), job security, and benefits. As Nadine always said, "This system will only work if it is ultimately a state project—if it is to be sustainable, it has to be run through the state." Since CASA established this path, Mujeres Aliadas school has also attained its RVOE.

Others, however, such as Nueve Lunas school in Oaxaca City, Oaxaca (described in Chapter 5), felt that women should have the option to be seen outside the formal system and worried that the fact that 96 percent of births took place in regional, state-run general hospitals was actually a problem: too many low-risk births were clogging up the system in these hospitals, which should be reserved for those with complications or risk factors. Some schools aimed to train midwives who would work independently of these hospital systems; with this goal in mind, securing state-sanctioned licensure for midwifery-school graduates was less of a priority because they would not be working in the state health-care system. This vision also drew from the recognition that many of the women in the communities that most needed midwives (because they had less access to services) may be the ones where educational levels were already lower; therefore, offering midwifery training that did not depend on a preset level of educational achievement made sense.

Another important piece of the debate around to what extent midwifery should be tied to the state had to do with the economics of care. On the one hand, state oversight and the institutionalization of midwifery training and of midwives working within the health-care system meant that patients could access them at low or no cost through public facilities. For patients, even though CASA's estimated 3,500-peso (about 280 US dollars) fee for a vaginal birth was at least half the cost of a birth with a private doctor,[10] it increasingly could not compete with the free birth services at the public hospital. This same cost concern arose with births attended by midwives from the other schools, as well as among traditional midwives, even though they often charged much less than CASA, for example. It also meant, as stated above, that the midwives themselves could receive a set salary from the government and that their education could be state funded.

CASA students cost the school 3,700 pesos a month to train (about 300 US dollars), though the students only paid a small amount, and the rest had to be made up for with private funding sources.

On the other hand, becoming a part of the state system means losing the kinds of flexibility and autonomy that many midwives and aspiring midwifery students envision as an integral part of the job. However, if such flexibility and autonomy come at a price—both for the students and the patients—some ask whether it is sustainable or, ultimately, just.

Over the years I spent at different midwifery schools across Mexico, I watched as midwives, students, and administrators debated the validity of their educational models. Their arguments drew on the factors described above—economic concerns, existing educational levels, and opportunities and problems with the health-care system. Yet they all shared basic principles about midwives' role in humanizing care for women. They wanted women to have choices and to be treated with respect, and they wanted to protect reproductive health care from the encroachment of overzealous medicalization, which they saw as frequently unnecessary and often dangerous or violent.

When new educational options came on the scene purporting to offer midwifery-style training within existing university-based nursing programs, many of the midwives were skeptical. Perinatal nurses and licensed obstetrical nurses (LEOs) are nurses with a specialization in obstetrics, and word was going around that the LEOs in particular were being seen by government officials as a better bet than trained midwives. LEOs have been around for decades, but it was not until recently that they were given more autonomy to work with women in labor (Atkin et al. 2019). Some LEOs were even referring to themselves as midwives, I was told. Many of the midwives I had worked with scoffed at the idea that nurses would compare themselves to midwives—saying that LEOs were far too medicalized from their nursing training and work experience in hospitals.

Midwives' disdain for the medicalized approach LEOs represented was part of their bigger set of concerns about the misuse of biomedical interventions. It seemed that, within the midwifery schools, the worst insult one student could make about another was to call her a *mini-médica* (mini-doctor); these students worried that LEOs would all be *mini-médicas*, because they were learning in hospital settings already steeped in biomedical approaches to women's health and reproduction. This was not just a dogmatic response to biomedicine and its institutions but rather the manifestation of real concerns about a lack of evidence-based practices.[11] Nadine argued that an investment in LEOs was not going to result in better care or better health outcomes. "The LEOs are caring people who think they are midwives, but they are not," she told me one afternoon as we talked on her patio. "They have such high C-section rates, which really goes to show, you know, that the proof is in the pudding." For Nadine, the highly medicalized approach of the LEOs stood in contrast with what CASA was trying to instill in its students: a humanized approach to birth that did not over-rely on medical intervention.

"Furthermore," Nadine continued, "many LEOs are from the upper or upper middle class, from urban areas, and they cannot relate to rural populations. They won't go to those areas; they won't help those people." While Nadine's comment does not necessarily account for the breadth of nursing students' backgrounds in Mexico,[12] it does point to a finding that the MacArthur Foundation's report also notes: neither nurses nor doctors are easy to recruit or retain in geographically marginalized regions of Mexico (like Guerrero, Puebla, or Veracruz), because of their location and lower salaries (Atkin et al. 2019, 42). This geography problem has persisted despite concerted state attempts to distribute practitioners across rural Mexico, such as through mandating social service for new graduates since the 1930s (Soto Laveaga 2013). All of the midwifery schools I studied emphasized the need to train students who would bring quality care to the regions of Mexico that had been historically marginalized. While LEOs may increase the number of skilled birth attendants in urban areas and hospital settings, what about the women who live in rural regions or who simply do not want to go to the hospital for their birth?

The schools I studied had different opinions about whether midwives should be working in the formal health-care system or building an autonomous system that offered more flexibility and choice to women and their providers. This debate echoed a larger debate the MacArthur Foundation found in their 2015–2018 analysis of Mexican midwifery, which concluded that with the rising interest in and options for midwifery in Mexico, "two distinct strategies or movements have emerged: the midwife as ideal provider for situations of normal birth versus promotion of evidence-based, women-centered maternal and neonatal care by all providers" (Atkin et al. 2019, 35). While many of the midwives I worked with argued that the former was correct—that is, that midwives were the experts in maternal health— the increasing state support for training nurses to attend births indicated that the state felt the second option more appropriate. Indeed, the 2017 National Center for Gender Equity and Reproductive Health (CNEGySR) proposal, "The Model for Professional Midwifery Services," which emphasized the incorporation of midwifery services into existing fields of obstetric and perinatal nursing, was welcomed by the health ministry as more viable than investing in midwifery as a separate profession (Atkin et al. 2019). This growing state support for midwifery as simply an add-on to nursing worried many of the midwives with whom I worked. At the very least, they argued, to meet the demand of women across Mexico's diverse regions, midwifery would need to remain diverse and not be confined only to nursing: there would need to be different types of midwives who could practice in different settings, to meet women where they are (geographically or culturally).

In any case, the consensus was that Mexico needed more trained midwives of one kind or another to really meet the demand that was overwhelming the current system. One recent report argues that, to improve health outcomes, Mexico should train at least 2,700 midwives so that they could attend at least 20 percent of the 2,400,000 annual births in Mexico; if Mexico were to fully institutionalize midwifery in the manner of countries like Peru or Chile, this number would have to be much higher (Faget and Capasso 2017).

Why Do Midwifery Students Think Midwives Matter in Mexico?

Midwifery students were being told that their country needed them. While they came into their studies with wide-ranging ideas about what midwives even were, their narrative about why the profession was so needed in Mexico began to coalesce as they progressed in their programs. It was nearly the end of the academic year when I surveyed midwifery students at CASA and Mujeres Aliadas schools and asked them why they thought midwifery mattered in Mexico (among other survey questions).[13] The results, shown in Figure 4, resonated with the messaging put forth by the then newly formed Asociación Mexicana de Partería (Mexican Midwifery Association) and by school administrators. By the end of their first year, students framed maternal mortality reduction as the primary reason that Mexico needed midwives, closely followed by the need to promote humanized or dignified birthing conditions. This dual emphasis was something that I saw reflected throughout my conversations with midwives. I argue that it reveals their politically savvy shift from emphasizing their fundamental goal (to improve the quality of care and treatment of women) to emphasizing the goal of maternal mortality reduction in order to resonate more explicitly with national and global health targets (a shift that is discussed in detail in Chapter 2).

The third most important reason given for the need for midwives was the idea that midwives help empower women by giving them information and options. Interestingly, this was an idea put forth only by more advanced CASA and Mujeres Aliadas students. As I discuss in this book's Conclusion, midwives developed a counter narrative to combat the ways they saw women being treated in the current health-care system: in their counter narrative, women became the protagonists and were empowered by having conditions that allowed them to make their own decisions regarding their care. It makes sense that only more advanced students saw this as a reason for Mexico to invest in midwifery; the idea of empowering women, of women becoming the protagonists of their own birth, is a more high-level analysis of the situation, requiring an understanding of how maternal conditions collide with opportunity and, ultimately, dictate health experiences and outcomes. Yet the message that female empowerment leads to better health outcomes was not invented by the midwives; they were joining a well-worn conversation that has been a major feature of global health policies that envision empowerment as the key to solving global poverty (Maes et al. 2015).

When, as I described above, Nadine gathered the first-year CASA students and told them that they were now part of a movement steeped in social justice and aimed at changing the system, many were confused about the relationship between systemic change and midwifery training. As they progressed through their education, however, they began to integrate what they were learning in the classroom and during clinical rotations with Nadine's messages of inequality, access, and political power. They began to see how what they were doing did go beyond helping individual women during pregnancy and birth and to view midwifery as something that had the potential to both empower women and address bigger issues that held political sway, like maternal and fetal mortality.

What was interesting was that, while Nadine had one vision of how this movement would be accomplished—largely through systemic change brought about by midwives working within the Mexican health-care system to change it—the students viewed their roles in the movement in a variety of ways. This diversity reflected their individual backgrounds, skills, and

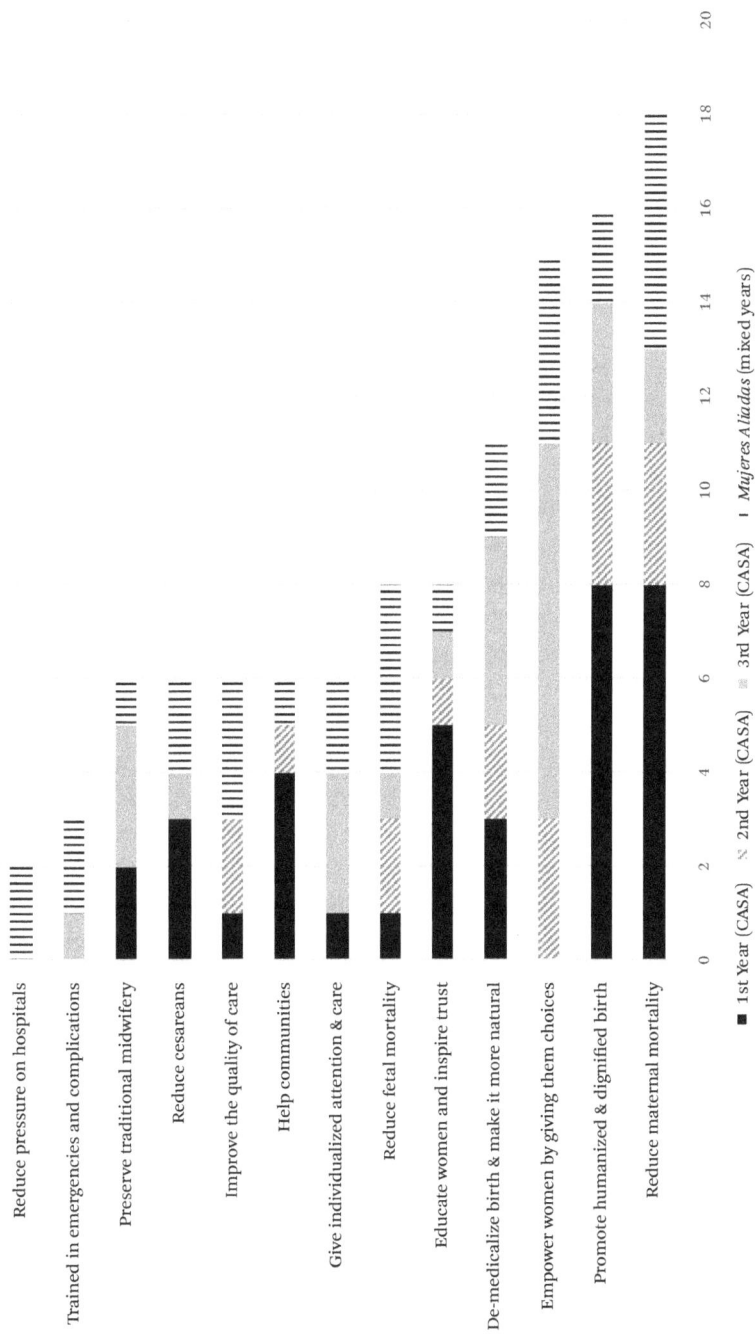

FIGURE 4: Midwifery student responses to survey about why midwifery is necessary in Mexico.

Reduce pressure on hospitals

Trained in emergencies and complications

Preserve traditional midwifery

Reduce cesareans

Improve the quality of care

Help communities

Give individualized attention & care

Reduce fetal mortality

Educate women and inspire trust

De-medicalize birth & make it more natural

Empower women by giving them choices

Promote humanized & dignified birth

Reduce maternal mortality

0   2   4   6   8   10   12   14   16   18   20

■ 1st Year (CASA)   ▨ 2nd Year (CASA)   ▨ 3rd Year (CASA)   ‖ Mujeres Aliadas (mixed years) career aspirations, and collectively it began to paint a picture of what midwifery was and could be in Mexico today and into the future.

One way that the students' visions diverged slightly from Nadine's was related to their career goals. In the same survey described above, I asked students where they planned to work once they completed their training. Of the thirty-six respondents, more than half (nineteen) echoed Nadine and Mujeres Aliadas' founder Diana's goals for them, stating that they planned to return to their own communities to care for the people there (the rest were unsure, planned to go wherever they were most needed, wanted to travel and learn from other practitioners before settling down, or wanted to remain near the school location). However, while Nadine felt that the best way to change women's health-care delivery was to certify midwives to allow them to create change from within the health-care system, most (twenty-four) students stated that they ultimately wanted to work out of a home setting.

I recently met up with two CASA alumni and was chatting with them about their experiences since they graduated. "Even after being in school together for three years, we all came away with such different ideas about what kind of midwife we wanted to be. Everyone has done such different things with their degrees," one of them told me. They described how some of their colleagues had gone on to work in state clinics or hospitals, one returned to Guatemala to bring professional midwifery there, and others got scooped up by NGOs hoping to improve health outcomes in rural regions across the country. The two I spoke with were back in San Miguel de Allende to see old friends. One of them had gone to work with another CASA alumna at a freestanding birth center, where they attended "women who are terrified to go to the hospital or women who just want a different kind of treatment." They included traditional Mexican and alternative medicine in their practice and had found a network of local doctors to serve as backup when needed. The other alumna had returned to her home country in South America, where she was starting to take on home-birth clients but dreamed of opening the country's first professional midwifery school to be able to train more midwives and reach more people.

Conclusion

When I talk to midwives around Mexico who have gone through the schools I studied, I sometimes get the sense that they are each a sort of drop in the

bucket—there are so many women in need of quality care and so few practicing midwives. CASA was no longer accepting students when I last went
to visit, though its model was being copied by various states, and the idea
of professional midwifery was gaining traction slowly. Nadine explained
to me that it was time, after developing the curriculum for professional
midwifery in Mexico and graduating 120 midwives, to reevaluate CASA's
model; for her, it had always been about trying to get the Mexican government to see the value of midwifery education. Now that some states were
finally replicating CASA's model, Nadine wanted to rethink what they, as an
NGO, should be doing.[14] Mujeres Aliadas had finally achieved the ability
to grant its graduates the *cédula profesional* so that they could practice in
state facilities, but they could only train so many students at a time. Nueve
Lunas did not offer any such certificate to its graduates and was also limited in the number of graduates it could produce.

But the evidence of their impact is increasingly woven throughout the
Mexican health-care system in ways that are not always immediately obvious.
I trace this evidence as I follow news stories, publications, and midwifery-
school graduates through their careers. Obstetric violence (discussed more
in Chapter 4) has become a talking point in the media and among academics, largely because of the midwives' lobbying to bring such violence to light.
In Guanajuato, the state where CASA's school was located, the state adopted
new paperwork for laboring women in public hospitals that explicitly asked
which *atención amigable* (friendly attention) procedures were carried out by
providers (for example, whether the woman was allowed to walk around,
given a massage during labor, used a birthing ball, etc.). In 2018, Mexico
passed a law stating that women were allowed to have a support person
with them during labor and delivery. While the combined effects of these
public acknowledgments of the need to change how women are treated in
labor may have not yet translated to radical shifts in actual practices (women
are not suddenly being treated differently or even allowed to have partners
in the labor ward, despite changes in forms and laws), they are important
steps in building conditions within which women have more choice and
support. And midwives have been behind them.

In a recent talk with Nadine, catching up about CASA and midwifery in
Mexico more generally, I asked her how she saw things "going" on a national
scale. "*Pues . . . allí vamos*" (Well, we're getting there), she said with a wry
chuckle. I laughed with her and said, "Maybe that is what I should title
this book—*Allí Vamos.*" She laughed with me, sighed, and said that they

had made progress, even if it was sometimes hard to see. But she wanted more. And she felt strongly, as always, that to build a better system, Mexico had to invest in midwifery in a real way. For Nadine, this meant supporting midwifery that embraced medical pluralism (drawing from biomedical and traditional or alternative practices) while avoiding overmedicalization or unnecessary interventions, trained students who could work in marginalized communities, and offered a viable educational and career path for young women to become care providers given Mexico's educational context.

Like the students whose survey results are discussed above, Nadine saw midwifery as something that could improve a range of issues related to social inequality. Their shared visions of the relationships between reproduction and inequality mirror the reproductive justice framework employed by academics and activists alike, which challenges outdated notions of reproductive rights by positing that health cannot be achieved without creating the conditions within which people can be healthy; without quality care available to all women, there is no "right" to health. What's more, the midwives I worked with shared "the reproductive justice paradigm's focus on marginalized communities," which "recognizes that women's reproductive rights are meaningless without addressing the social contexts in which these rights are exercised, including historically oppressive structures of racial, economic, and sexual inequality" (Gurr 2014, 33).

Over the years I became familiar with midwives' narratives about the potential for midwifery to bridge the divide between a broken health-care system, a population of people whose trust in that system had eroded, and a government who needed to improve outcomes to meet its own targets. In the next chapter, I look specifically at how Mexican midwives are navigating national and global discourse around maternal mortality reduction as the primary focus of development initiatives in reproductive health. Through this navigation, they maintain their middle ground, operating in sync with this discourse while simultaneously challenging its assumptions and pushing for the expanded scope of what counts when it comes to women's bodies and experiences.

CHAPTER 2

Breaking Out of the "Uterus Box"

Like the CASA school described in previous chapters, Mujeres Aliadas (Allied Women)—located just outside Pátzcuaro, Michoacán—aimed to produce what it called "professional midwives." Diana was a certified nurse midwife from Chicago whose work with patients originating from Michoacán ultimately inspired her to move there with her husband, Brian, an epidemiologist, and co-found the midwifery school in February 2011.[1] They had begun work in the area some years before, during which time they assessed the needs of the communities surrounding the lake of Pátzcuaro, a region where many Indigenous Purépecha people live. Based on their assessment, they decided to build their organization with three prongs—the midwifery school, the clinic, and a peer-educator program. Each of these prongs addresses what they found to be the primary needs of the local population, though from different angles: the school trains local women to have sustainable and meaningful employment helping other women and families, the clinic gives women a place to go for humane and holistic women's healthcare needs, and the peer educators are able to bring information into the communities that can help change behaviors and offer a bridge to services where barriers exist. By the time I arrived at Mujeres Aliadas, they had been in operation for a year. They had built a functioning peer-education model working in the communities, opened a clinic that served local residents and established opportunities to conduct short-term outreach projects through state clinics, and tailored their vision for the school's goals and future in response to early experiences: it was now more clearly aimed at training rural nurses to become midwives who could work in local clinics or in stand-alone birth centers.

Getting to Pátzcuaro by bus entailed a stunning ride through a region of Mexico that people often told me was one of the nation's most beautiful—although when I first went in February 2011, many also warned me that it had become one of the most dangerous as well. Stories of hijacked cars and roadside theft were common there, although my own trip was smooth and easy. I arrived in the town of Pátzcuaro in the early afternoon during a torrential downpour and stood huddling under a small shelter until Brian picked me up. "Look for the South Dakota license plates," he had told me when we arranged this meeting by email. Later he explained that a lot of ex-pats used South Dakota plates, which you could order online without having to go back to the United States. Brian took me by their home, a lovely adobe-style house with a view of the town and the surrounding hills, to pick up Diana before heading to the school site.

Mujeres Aliadas surprised me with its beauty—it felt more like a retreat than a school or clinic. It was located across Lake Pátzcuaro from the main town of Pátzcuaro, in the small and lovely village of Erongarícuaro (where, Diana told me later, Frida Kahlo and her counterculture comrades used to hang out). The school was housed in a small, rectangular building with glass windows all along one side that faced a green misty valley. Gardens surrounded the school building, and around the perimeter were a series of clinical rooms for women to be seen for checkups or births, housed in a building that matched the regional style of white walls and red-tiled roofs. Within these rooms medical equipment and hospital beds butted up alongside cozy, hand-carved wooden beds, painted in whimsical colors and laden with piles of woven blankets.

After I took in the beautiful surroundings, Diana and Brian began asking me questions about midwifery in other parts of Mexico. I knew that Mujeres Aliadas had connections with some of the other schools, but they were eager for my perspective on how things were going in general for midwifery and specifically in the other schools that I had been working with. Diana, like the administrators of all of the schools I studied, was looking for the right path to make her school viable. While CASA was still widely seen as the most established program, and had already forged some of the pathways toward legitimacy, it was always unclear to what degree CASA's path could be replicated in other settings or whether it would be possible to carve a slightly different path and still attain similar state recognition. Diana's vision was similar to CASA founder Nadine's in some ways (and indeed, after completing my fieldwork I would learn that Mujeres Aliadas students were finally allowed to apply for the *cédula profesional*—the professional, federally recognized license to practice that CASA had created), yet her motivation for and pedagogical design around the Mujeres Aliadas midwifery school came from a very different place.

"Our main focus here is on gynecology," Diana told me emphatically that first afternoon. I wasn't expecting this, as gynecological training was not very strong at CASA, where I had spent most of my time with students thus far. CASA students were taught to identify and treat basic gynecological issues, but as a focus of study it was secondary to the issues around primary care in pregnancy and birth. For Diana, this was a huge mistake. "The lack of focus on gynecological issues in other training programs is a big problem," she argued. For her, midwifery was about caring for a woman's health throughout her life, not just during pregnancy and childbirth, and gynecological issues such as bacterial vaginal infections and sexually transmitted diseases were within the midwives' scope of practice. Furthermore, Diana had witnessed the rampant undiagnosed or misdiagnosis of such diseases and infections in this region. "That has been the single biggest health problem that we have encountered in the communities where we work," she told me. Mujeres Aliadas was created in the hopes of offering a new kind of practitioner who could work in the communities and in the clinics but who could also bring renewed attention to gynecological issues faced by many women there. Diana saw the lack of standardized training in gynecological diagnosis and treatment as a huge failing of the existing midwifery training programs.

In order to have access to clinical positions for graduating students—an issue that CASA has solved by securing the cédula profesional for its graduates so that they could work in state facilities—Mujeres Aliadas had become a school for nurses. That is, all of the students there were already licensed nurses, and thus already had access to work within clinics. Diana's hope was that they would continue to have such access once they were trained as midwives, as well, although the organization was also working hard to secure their own cédulas for the graduates. While this arrangement of training nurses may have facilitated their acceptance within established medical settings, Diana admitted that they hadn't actually started out with that plan in mind. In fact, their original class had many students in it who were not nurses but still wanted to be midwives. Ultimately, Diana realized that those who had not already studied nursing simply couldn't keep up with the materials, and they all had to leave the program.

A class made up completely of trained nurses fit well into Diana's vision for a midwifery practice which took gynecological problems as seriously as pregnancy and birth; nurses already understood gynecological diseases and were familiar with the procedures for testing and treating these diseases. It was much easier to work with students who already had these skills, Diana told me. She noted that two of her primary staff midwives—who had been, interestingly, hired after they finished their degrees at CASA—proved competent in labor care but had very little understanding of gynecological issues. She argued that if her students already had a background in nursing, they would be able to manage women's health concerns throughout their life cycles.

This approach made sense to Diana in large part, I realized, because of her own training and background as a certified nurse midwife from the United States. While CASA's Nadine brought with her a background in public health and social work and ultimately focused on broader issues of social justice, Diana brought her nurse midwifery training to her focus on comprehensive patient care. The founders of Nueve Lunas school (discussed more in Chapter 5) brought yet another perspective to midwifery education—that of traditionally trained midwives focusing on the preservation of local skills as a way to help marginalized regions maintain tradition and access to care.

What all of these schools shared, and what I examine through this chapter, was an ability to frame their diverse approaches to midwifery training and care in relationship to—rather than in spite of—the universalizing attempts of global health policies. This argument extends our understanding of the relationship between grassroots health projects and global health initiatives. Specific, measurable outcomes have increasingly come to define what matters in health on both the local and global scales (Adams 2016). The target that has emerged as the primary motivator for development in the field of women's health in Mexico, as globally, is maternal mortality reduction. The research into the effects of these patterns in the field of women's health has shown the ways that the emphasis on a universal reduction in maternal mortality metrics gets in the way of really understanding women's needs and experiences in diverse contexts (Wendland 2016; Oni-Orisan 2016).

I agree that the push toward universals and accountability on every level—local, national, and global—to achieve universal numerical targets for health, including maternal mortality ratios, does all of those things. This is a phenomenon of growing importance, as we see more and more health interventions framed in direct and sometimes myopic response to such targets. Indeed, a historical view of universal metrics in global health reveals a legacy of enforced cooperation with global targets, especially among postcolonial populations, in which ideas of universality and objectivity "had to be taught and learned and forged in a crucible of colonial occupations" (Adams 2016, 20). Ethnographic inquiry can be a powerful tool to trace the relationships between global targets, ideas of universality, and local practices. By observing midwives at work and talking to midwives and politicians alike about what matters in women's health care in Mexico, I was able to see how, on the one hand, the push for standardization was marginalizing practitioners and, sometimes, reducing women's options for care in settings where their access had already been historically constricted.

But I also argue that ethnographic engagement with the providers and educators on the ground allows us to see these universalizing attempts in a different light: the midwives and midwifery schools examined in this book stand as examples of those who see the effects of these metrics and have found ways to work with them to their advantage.

In this chapter, I show how the midwives at Mujeres Aliadas came to see the impacts of the narrowly focused, numbers-based approach to women's health through the bodies and experiences of their patients. I also describe how they used the language and goals of global health targets to justify their own work, while continuing to engage in grass-roots training and care that departed from the one-size-fits-all approach imagined in universalizing global health interventions. The midwives featured in this chapter, as throughout this book, were strategic. They learned that their outward messaging must be flexible enough to conform to the expectations passed down by global health policies and that their goals for health outcomes must align with those laid out by universal targets. But they also learned that, if they could pitch themselves in ways that development agencies understood and cared about (as tools for maternal mortality reduction), they might just be able to keep working on building a model of care that addressed the issues not covered in global health policies: they could reduce the poor outcomes that had not been put into clear, universal targets while continuing to champion their patients and communities. The research has largely supported the midwives' claims that their presence could reduce maternal deaths.

Why women die before, during, or after childbirth is a complicated question, the answer to which is necessarily connected to both underlying health issues and structural issues related to access to and quality of care. More than half of maternal deaths worldwide are attributed to hypertensive disorders, hemorrhage, and sepsis (Say et al. 2014). With prenatal care, trained birth attendants, and comprehensive postpartum care, most of these deaths could be avoided. In Mexico, as in many countries, maternal deaths resulting from these primary kinds of causes—termed "direct maternal deaths"—did decline significantly between 2006 and 2013 (Hogan et al. 2016). Yet maternal deaths resulting from *indirect* causes (linked to pre-existing conditions such as HIV, mental health disorders, or diabetes) remained constant during that time period. As chronic health conditions such as HIV, diabetes, and mental health disorders become more common worldwide, and in the absence of sufficient health care to address them, how will maternal mortality rates fare? Hogan et al. (2016) urge Mexico to invest not only in trained birth attendants, but also in comprehensive prenatal and postpartum care, with providers trained to recognize risk signs and treat underlying conditions before they manifest as emergencies or lead to fatality.

The WHO recognizes that reducing maternal mortality is not only about getting women into hospitals for childbirth and that any approach must be holistic and responsive to social needs as well as medical needs. It lists poverty, distance to facilities, a lack of information, poor quality or inadequate services, and cultural beliefs as the primary factors that stand in the way of women receiving good care during pregnancy and beyond (WHO n.d.). Women's dying during or soon after childbirth is not *only* a result of a lack of resources or access to competent care, though these are problems that Mexican midwives explicitly offer to help address.

Indeed, if the underlying causes of maternal death are to be adequately addressed, women need access to providers who can "treat the entire woman and not just her pregnancy" (Hogan et al. 2016, 366); that is, they need providers who can understand, diagnose, and address the indirect causes of death, as well as the social conditions in which the woman lives.

Midwives like Diana's claims to address maternal mortality alongside a host of other health issues are rooted in their ideas about how to change maternal conditions. Not only do they want to offer comprehensive care that recognizes women's myriad health-care needs, but they also want to make it clear that such a model for care could begin to address poor conditions by giving women choice, respect, and dignity.

Testing the System

Diana's training did not fully prepare her for all of the kinds of knowledge she and her students would need in order to provide such comprehensive care. While I visited her, she was in the midst of trying to learn, along with her students, how to perform their own lab tests for patients. This was for Diana another important element of gynecological care—being able to offer reliable, standardized lab results and thus treat women with the correct intervention. The topic of lab tests and their current lack of standardization came up one evening as we headed to dinner to talk more about Mujeres Aliadas.

We had left the school for the day and were driving back toward downtown Pátzcuaro when Diana suddenly stopped the car and rolled down her window, motioning to a passing woman to come closer. The woman clearly knew Diana and smiled as she approached. "Have you gotten your test results yet?" Diana asked her. "Not yet—on Wednesday!" the woman said. They said goodbye, and we drove off, the woman heading down a side street. Because Diana regularly assisted her students in their midwifery clinic outside town, I assumed that the woman was a regular patient of hers and didn't think much of the exchange.

However, after we had driven a few blocks, Diana began to tell the woman's story, explaining her urgency in wanting to know about her lab results. The woman had come to their clinic and told Diana that she belonged to IMSS Oportunidades (Mexico's conditional cash transfer program that was started in the 1990s under the name Progresa, most recently known as Prospera, and cut from the budget in 2019) and that five years ago she had gotten her pap test done as part of her required yearly Oportunidades checkup. Pap tests were just one of the medical routines necessary to receive the cash benefits of the Oportunidades program. The test she did then took weeks to be evaluated; she did not get the results back until she was already twenty weeks pregnant. When she was finally given the results, they said that she had stage three cervical cancer and sent her to a specialist. The specialist told her that the only choice was to abort the fetus and do a hysterectomy. The woman left the office devastated about the diagnosis and proposed treatment. After talking to her family, she ultimately chose not to comply with the recommendations and gave birth to a healthy baby a few months later. That was five years ago, and she had not been back for another pap test since.

When the woman arrived at the Mujeres Aliadas clinic and told Diana her story, Diana immediately sent her pap into a private local lab in order to get the results faster (the state labs, Diana explained, were infamous for taking months to return results). The results indicated that the patient only had vaginitis, a common and, if treated, non-serious diagnosis of vaginal inflammation that could signal bacterial vaginosis, trichomoniasis, or a yeast infection. Diana commented that she had actually never seen a patient's pap result in this area *not* show up positive for vaginitis; it was extremely common and frequently went untreated for months or years. It was also not something women were unaware of as a problem, they just did not always know what to do about their symptoms, how to get help, or how to follow up when their treatment did not work or their symptoms reoccurred. Indeed, when I was chatting with one of Mujeres Aliadas' peer educators, she told me, "I love giving *platicas* (talks) in the communities on all kinds of topics, but the women always want to know about vaginal infections more than anything else!" Mujeres Aliadas spent a large part of its budget giving free medications to women with these chronic infections. So, when the results came back as positive for vaginitis, Diana and the patient were both confused, though relieved, to get a result that conflicted so seriously with the previous stage three cervical cancer result. They initially assumed that the original test had been wrong, and that this more common result was indeed the correct one.

Diana's relief was short-lived, however; because of the woman's history, Diana advised her to re-test in three months. Again, her test came back from the private lab saying that she had nothing serious. Soon after, however, the woman returned to her Oportunidades clinic for another pap test in order to receive her next conditional cash transfer. This pap came back notifying her once again that she had stage three cervical cancer.

Diana was devastated that her own private lab had given such different and conclusively benign results for her patient. She confronted the lab personnel, who argued that they had the best equipment and most up-to-date training. They told her that they could not have made a mistake. The patient was, by this point, obviously upset and confused about the differing diagnoses. Oportunidades sent her for a biopsy, the results of which were what Diana was asking her about that day on the street.

Shaken by this experience, Diana decided to conduct an experiment of her own. She had her midwifery students collect two identical samples from a patient during a gynecological exam. They sent the samples to two different labs that they had used in the past. One test was sent back saying that the woman had five different infections; the other came back saying that the woman had zero. This discrepancy further confirmed Diana's growing suspicion that women were not being correctly diagnosed or treated for gynecological issues.

Diana was not the first to notice inconsistencies in pap test results in Mexico. Pap tests are conducted to look for changes in the cervix that could indicate cancerous or precancerous cells. Cervical cancer is the second leading cause of cancer deaths in Mexican women, despite being highly curable if detected early through pap testing (Unger-Saldaña, Alvarez-Meneses, and Isla-Ortiz 2018). The government did begin a national cervical cancer screening program in 1974 in the hopes of systematically addressing this concern (Sankaranarayanan, Madhukar Budukh, and Rajkumar 2001). However, a study reviewing the quality of pap test laboratory readings in Mexico City found a false negative prevalence that was at least triple the prevalence found in industrialized countries (Lazcano-Ponce et al. 1994, 13); false negatives occur in around 35 percent of specimens (Garcia et al. 2003, 471). In a country with such high rates of cervical cancer, these false negatives are very concerning; women who could benefit from early intervention, and who comply with state testing programs, are being sent on their way thinking that they have nothing to worry about. How could this happen? Studies have pointed to multiple aspects of testing that can go wrong for women to end up with an incorrect result, as when samples are not taken or processed correctly or information on patients' age, health history, and symptoms are not included with the sample (details that are important for helping determine diagnoses) (Lazcano-Ponce et al. 1994, 13). These inconsistencies in the quality of laboratory results, coupled with low screening rates and a lack of gynecological care (especially for the most marginalized and at-risk parts of the population), have been shown through multiple studies to explain why Mexico has struggled to reduce cervical cancer rates (Unger-Saldaña, Alvarez-Meneses, and Isla-Ortiz 2018; Garcia et al. 2003).

Diana was not solely interested in testing for and preventing cervical cancer, however. When she told me that Mujeres Aliadas' main focus was on gynecological health, she meant all aspects of gynecological health. Maternal mortality continues to be the primary motivator for health interventions related to women, and cervical cancer prevention has drawn up as a close second as a preventable and measurable indicator of national health. While those are both important campaigns to support, Diana's argument was that women suffer from many other gynecological conditions that negatively affect their lives but may not get as much attention because they do not end in measurable deaths. This burden of gynecological health problems falls disproportionately on marginalized populations in Mexico, as elsewhere:

for example, 85 percent of all women who die from cervical cancer are in the developing world (Robinson, Stoffel, and Haider 2015, 211).

As Diana and her colleagues tried to bring attention to women's health beyond their reproductive processes, they were attempting to expand the category of women's health within a global framework that had become increasingly narrow in its scope of interest, despite evidence showing the damage such narrowing can cause. Within resource-poor settings worldwide, women's health efforts focus primarily on prenatal and obstetric care, even as issues related to sexually transmitted infections (STIs), urogynecologic conditions like fistulas or pelvic organ prolapse, and family planning concerns have a significant impact on women's health outcomes: for example, STIs, if left untreated, can lead to a host of chronic and debilitating diseases and symptoms that decrease women's health and have potential impacts on their pregnancies, as well (Robinson, Stoffel, and Haider 2015). Even the extremely frequent vaginitis results Diana had seen revealed a fundamental failure in the health-care system, for while vaginitis may generally be treatable and not sound as serious as cervical cancer or maternal mortality, it still can lead to a host of other health issues ranging in severity from increased risk of STIs to preterm labor (Chavoustie et al. 2017), not to mention discomfort, self-esteem issues, and embarrassment. If women were not getting testing and treatment for a full range of gynecological concerns elsewhere, Diana wanted to make sure that Mujeres Aliadas could fill the need.

Her solution had been, so far, to try to teach her students to read lab tests themselves using equipment, like microscopes, in their clinic. "The only thing I don't know how to teach them is to test for chlamydia," she said, "but I know we can learn." For Diana, being able to teach her students to read their own lab tests had thus become imperative, as she could no longer trust the expertise of the established laboratories. This mistrust in laboratories fits into the broader infrastructure failures discussed in Chapter 3; when practitioners and patients cannot trust the results of their studies, they may give or receive incorrect or inadequate treatment. It also reflects the kind of improvisational skills necessary when practicing health care at the margins (Wendland 2010; Livingston 2012).

At Mujeres Aliadas, being able to do one's own lab testing was framed as a way to improve upon the biomedical system, empower practitioners, and offer higher quality of care to patients. It also seemed possible only because of Diana's training as a nurse practitioner and her students' prior training. CASA's students were directed to rely on specialists to do things like read lab tests, as they were trained from the start to work within the existing health-care system and as the scope of their own training was not wide enough to encompass laboratory skills. For Diana, it was not enough to rely on an uncertain existing infrastructure of biomedicine—her students must be able to act autonomously and rely on themselves and each other to offer the best possible care. This emphasis on self-reliant midwives that could diagnose and treat women for a large range of gynecological and reproductive health issues formed the backbone of Mujeres Aliadas' mission. For Diana, midwives needed to care for women throughout their lives, not just in the moment of reproduction.

This more holistic emphasis on women's reproductive health, however, was not what was motivating the larger political reevaluation of midwives; maternal mortality was still a concept concerned primarily with preventing maternal death in the moment of reproduction, not improving women's health overall. Diana had not been the first person involved in women's health in Mexico to mention the role maternal mortality reduction campaigns were having in shaping opportunities and constraints for care. I soon came to realize that the history behind—and contemporary projects around—maternal mortality reduction in Mexico were key to understanding how midwives fit into today's health-care system.

The Rise and Fall and Stagnation of Maternal Mortality in Mexico

Maternal mortality—*mortalidad materna*—was a topic on the tip of everyone's tongue throughout my fieldwork. This was not the case when I first began working with midwives in Mexico in 2002, then as a volunteer intern who was getting to know many of the midwives I would ultimately work with throughout my research. At that time, the midwives I worked with were more likely to speak of the importance of *el parto humanizado* (humanized birth) or *el parto respetado* (respected birth), by which they meant a model of birth that treated women with dignity and respect. Maternal mortality, which refers to the number of women who die for every 100,000 live births, was a metric used by policy-makers—not something that the midwives were explicitly making claims to address. Yet over the years, I saw a marked change in the way that maternal mortality was discussed and operationalized by midwives across Mexico.

While humanizing birth was still the primary mission of the midwives I worked with, by 2009, maternal mortality had become the key term with which midwives were able to communicate with state officials. The emphasis on maternal mortality reduction is part of a larger set of what Dána-Ain Davis (2019, 121) calls "technologies of saving"—the interventions and policies that emerge in response to a need to save lives. Davis points out that the paradox of such saving technologies is that they become profitable and thus fixed, as whole industries arise to carry them out. Resources go toward saving lives rather than addressing prevention and dealing with the causes that lead to death in the first place. Mexican policy makers and government officials wanted to show that they were saving women and babies; a noble goal, obviously, but also one that offered better optics than preventative projects, which were perceived as less urgent. Midwives were savvy to the weight that promising maternal mortality reduction carried for their local and national policy makers, and they felt strongly that they offered a unique approach that could at once improve women's health care and secure a future for institutionalized midwifery.

So how did maternal mortality become such a central issue nationwide for midwives and policy makers alike? The history of its ascension to such a visible and politically motivating data point is important to understand, for while the reduction of maternal deaths is indeed a goal universally shared by midwives and policy makers alike, many feel that the primary emphasis on maternal mortality has eclipsed other pressing health concerns and simplified complex connections between underlying structural inequalities and individual women's health experiences and outcomes.

Throughout the brief history that follows regarding the development of maternal mortality reduction as a central state focus in Mexico, I maintain that the whittling down of global health initiatives regarding women to maternal death as a key indicator has resulted in a health-care infrastructure that is riddled with holes—the kinds of holes that Mujeres Aliadas' students were training to address. These holes in the system reflect the gaps in attention to things that midwives see as vital but that have not always received state, national, or global attention: things like comprehensive gynecological health care or humane treatment in birth.

Mexico's approach to maternal mortality reduction has been shaped by a series of global conferences and initiatives that have set the tone for national, state, and local priorities and have set in motion practices and procedures that directly affect women. It is important to remember that, as I describe in the Introduction, these global conferences and initiatives were built on the premise of Mexico as a developing country, a concept I recognize as problematic. Yet notions of development and modernization shaped the kinds of interventions that were applied in Mexico, as elsewhere, despite their opaque nature. The first call to action on a global scale related to reproduction was the First World Population Conference, held in Rome in 1954 by the United Nations, which called for more accurate demographic information of developing countries in order to understand population concerns. This was followed in 1965 by the Second World Population Conference in Belgrade, where fertility analysis was put on the policy agenda for development planning. The Third World Population Conference, held in 1974 in Bucharest, was where population policies were reframed as interdependent with all other socio-economic development concerns, an important step in the conceptualization of reproduction and reproductive health within a broader social context. This emphasis on context became more nuanced at the International Conference on Population and Development in Cairo in 1994, where women's reproductive health was for the first time framed as a human rights concern to the international sphere (Mayhew, Douthwaite, and Hammer 2006). While Cairo was an important turning point in the global framing of reproduction—not only because it stressed women's reproductive rights as vital to improving women's health outcomes but also because it reached a consensus that such rights are vital to all other markers of development, from education to nutrition to economic development— more recent international agendas retain little of the rights-based approach that was heralded as so revolutionary there (Crossette 2005).

By the time of the 1994 conference in Cairo, then, population had long been understood in the international sphere to be fully entangled with all other development policies. Cairo highlighted the need to view population issues as human rights concerns, not as stand-alone development goals (see UN 1995).[2] By the mid-nineties, reproductive health and sexual health were discussed as rights—rights that were vital to any projects of development.

After the Cairo meeting, Mexico joined other nations in signing on to reduce the focus on population control and instead "promote the integration of reproductive health services, such as counseling and testing for sexually transmitted infections during a woman's visit to a family planning clinic, or providing contraceptives to women after childbirth or an abortion" (A. Castro 2004, 133). Yet as Arachu Castro discovered, Mexican practitioners and politicians have not yet been able to get away from demographic targets as social goals, and so reproductive health practices are still shaped by such targets. The Mexican government created the Program on Reproductive Health and Family Planning in order to realign Mexican health policy with the international women's health movement that the conference had made cohesive and globally recognized. While Mexico was one of the first Latin American countries to engage with family planning programs through adopting official policies around the issue in the 1960s, it began by mostly carrying out its programs through sterilization and IUD insertion (A. Castro 2004). These two methods continue to be the most commonly used family planning methods (CONAPO 2016). While studies do indicate that the immediate postpartum insertion of IUDs can be an effective model for practitioners to follow to ensure contraceptive uptake (Lopez et al. 2015), the process for obtaining informed consent during active labor was questionable. I met many women who had tubal ligations, IUD insertions, or even hysterectomies immediately following their labor and were either completely unaware that the procedure had been done on them or were confused about what it meant and why it had been done (see Chapter 4 for a discussion of this phenomenon). Aside from the obvious ethical problems involved in forcibly sterilizing populations, these procedures cause women to incur further complications such as IUDs that are not inserted properly or complications from surgery, which were not addressed because of a lack of information.

These kinds of procedures are sticky, in that they stick around even after their value has been institutionally questioned. Doctors would tell me, "I learned to do things this way, so even though I know that the studies say not to, it is hard for me not to do things the way I learned them." While the doctors I spoke with believed that coercive sterilizations and IUD insertions were largely a thing of the past, they conceded that the mentality from those days prevailed among many of their colleagues: targets had to be met, and what women wanted was sometimes seen as secondary. When the next major global initiative to address reproductive health was crafted in 2000, the United Nations' Millennium Development Goals (MDGs), its structure dovetailed nicely with the direction in which Mexico was already heading: a numbers-based approach to health care that did not have to account for social inequalities.

The MDGs could have built off of Cairo's original framework of reproductive and sexual rights; instead, they delegated women's health to its previous status as an independent variable that did not depend on social and economic indicators. A major force behind this reversal in attitudes toward women's health was the opposition from the developing nations themselves, which was made up of many conservative members who did not support the language of the Cairo Program of Action in discussions of reproductive rights (Crossette 2005). As Sarah Williams puts it, the emphasis on "maternal health" as the sole aspect of women's health that mattered was "a politically and religiously palatable focus in reproductive health" (2019, 2). The MDGs came out of the Millennium Declaration, a document created by the United Nations, which had no direct reference to reproductive health or rights. When the goals were crafted, supporters of the Cairo consensus tried to change the language about "maternal health" to "reproductive health," but such changes were rejected—thus maintaining the focus on women's bodies as numerical indicators and not on women as individuals with the right to make decisions about their own lives and bodies (Crossette 2005).

The fifth MDG most clearly echoes the Cairo consensus, as it aimed to reduce maternal mortality by 75 percent between 1990 and 2015 and also increase access to reproductive health care (this secondary goal of reproductive health-care access was added later and has received less attention). The WHO defines maternal mortality as "the death of a woman while pregnant or within forty-two days of termination of pregnancy, irrespective of the duration and site of the pregnancy, from any cause related to or aggravated by the pregnancy or its management but not from accidental or incidental causes" (WHO 2014).

Of all of the concerns covered in the MDGs, maternal mortality makes a particularly significant indicator of development. For example, while infant mortality may be nearly ten times higher in developing countries than in developed countries, maternal mortality may rise to more than one hundred times higher in developing countries (Maine et al. 1997). Yet such distinctions cannot be solely tied to economic differences; while economic differences *have* been known for years to relate to differences in maternal mortality ratios between populations (McCarthy and Maine 1992), ethnic, racial, and individual characteristics including marital status are also important (Ronsmans and Graham 2006). The two principal causes of maternal death in Mexico—hypertension and hemorrhage—are in most cases preventable if treated correctly; in fact, the majority of maternal mortality cases are considered preventable. During the time I conducted this research, Mexican maternal mortality had declined somewhat in recent years—in 1990 there were 61 deaths per 100,000 live births, while in 2010 there were 51.5 deaths per 100,000 live births (Fernandez Canton, Gutierrez Trujillo, and Viguri

Uribe 2012). However, this number needed to decline further, and faster, if it was to reach the MDG's target. For Mexico, MDG number five meant that the country must lower its maternal mortality ratio to less than 22 deaths per 100,000 live births (Freyermuth and Sesia 2009).

Critics of the MDGs from both the international community and the Mexican midwifery community argued that Mexico would not come close to its target maternal mortality ratio unless it addressed social inequalities that were rendered invisible in the language of the development discourse. For example, Barbara Crossette argued that there is "nothing in the Millennium Development Goals about the fundamental physical hurdles women encounter starting within the family, often the extended family, where, in line with cultural practices, the woman may be treated as the property of male relatives or where in-laws may assert control to the point of violence against a young wife brought into the household" (2005, 75).

The midwives I worked with stressed that the MDGs also ignored inequalities related to race, ethnicity, and rural / urban divides across Mexico—maternal mortality in the relatively poorer state of Oaxaca, for example, is four times that of the wealthier state of Tlaxcala (Gómez Dantés et al. 2011, S222). Instead, they said, the narrow focus on maternal mortality had led to narrow solutions that rendered invisible such inequalities in favor of a strategy built on medicalization: Mexico had been steadily working toward getting all women to birth in hospitals, not at home or with midwives. As CASA founder Nadine told me, the MDGs and this focus on medicalization as the route to better health outcomes only served to "put women right back into the uterus box." By this, she meant that despite positive steps toward policies that focused on integrated women's health and equality, the MDGs had brought the emphasis back to women's bodies—and women's reproductive organs in particular. I titled this chapter using Nadine's quote because it was and is a striking visual: that a woman matters only when considering the reproductive potential of her uterus.

In Mexico, this focus on reproduction and emphasis on maternal mortality reduction resulted in the intensification of efforts to medicalize reproductive processes and bring birth into hospitals. Moving birth out of the home and into the hospital was and continues to be framed as a key strategy in preventing complications in birth (as it has been since the nineteenth century; see Chapter 1 for a discussion of this history). However, a paradox that midwives pointed out is that maternal mortality has not decreased significantly in recent years, despite the increase in births attended at hospitals.

For example, Mexico's cesarean rate is 46 percent (although it is higher in private hospitals—sometimes nearer to 80 or even 90 percent), putting it among the world's highest, yet its maternal mortality ratio remains high for its level of development (Alonso and Gerard 2009; Sesia 2017). That is significant because studies have shown that most cesarean sections performed are actually not indicated (the WHO [2015b] states that 10 to 15 percent is the acceptable rate for cesareans, though new research indicates that rates of above 10 percent at the population level may not show any effect on maternal and newborn mortality) and that, conversely, many women whose lives may have been saved by cesarean births are not receiving them. In this way, maternal mortality is also an interesting phenomenon in that it is a symptom both of over-medicalization *and* a lack of care and resources. It is therefore important to evaluate the motivations behind policies that target maternal mortality by either increasing the use of medical interventions in reproduction or, conversely, by decreasing their use. How maternal mortality is framed has important implications for how it is managed. The management of maternal mortality has various implications, in turn, for how women's bodies are managed.

Nadine's evocation of a "uterus box" in which women are stuck illustrates the concept of reproductive governance that scholars have increasingly described as a mechanism for surveillance and control (Williams 2019; Morgan and Roberts 2012). Reproductive governance has been a useful analytical tool with which to understand how global health policies, like the MDGs, interact with national interests and local infrastructures to shape reproductive choices and experiences. Key to this analysis is the notion that reproductive governance employs the use of moral regimes to enforce compliance with state or global health norms and policies. In Mexico, there has been a concerted effort to change reproductive health care-seeking behavior through morality. When women are told by health-care workers that they must abandon their midwives because they could endanger the lives of their children (a scenario women and midwives alike repeatedly described to me), they are being taught that, to be good parents and citizens, they need to rethink their relationship to the health-care system.

My findings were consistent with Williams, who found that "the moral regime of maternal health in Mexico holds that to be good mothers, women must give birth under the care of medical experts, and that emerging alive from this event is what constitutes a 'good birth.'" Williams goes on to argue that this moral regime stretches to the midwives themselves, dictating how they should practice if they are to align themselves with global development goals. She says that "the moral regime evinced by doctors in the Ministry of Health promotes the idea that in order for Indigenous women to be good midwives and support the imperative to lower MMR [maternal mortality rates], they must not practice midwifery" (2019, 7). Yet the midwives I worked with turned this messaging on its head and used it to argue that they were indeed more necessary now than ever to help the country achieve global health targets.

The target year of the MDGs, 2015, came and went, and Mexico—like many other countries—had not reached its goals for maternal mortality reduction (Rodríguez-Aguilar 2018). To the midwives I worked with, this did not really come as a surprise—they understood that the numbers would not drop to the levels required without a more holistic overhaul of the healthcare system and the ways women were treated within it. What did come as a surprise is that the midwives' perspective was echoed across the globe to such a degree that, when the WHO came back together to evaluate the terms of the MDGs and create the next set of goals—the Sustainable Development Goals (SDGs), meant to carry the world to 2030—they approached women's health very differently. They situated maternal mortality reduction as one of many intertwined health goals. The SDGs in general were much more exhaustive and represented a clear shift in thinking away from the idea that global development could be achieved through the improvement of a few key indicators and toward a recognition that there were many more issues in need of attention.

Despite being built into this more expansive framework, maternal mortality reduction was still highlighted as a key indicator for development; the SDGs laid out a global "average" target of less than 70 maternal deaths per 100,000 live births, as well as a goal for no individual nation to have a maternal mortality ratio greater than 140 (WHO 2015a, 83). These new targets explicitly emphasized a push to end *preventable* maternal deaths—a wording that brings to light the historical inadequacies that have allowed preventable deaths to go un-prevented, while framing the challenge as one that is also potentially achievable. If we name something as already preventable, we can prevent it, right?

Yet critics were quick to point out that the SDGs continued to provide elusive targets for change, even when addressing preventable causes of death. This was because the causes behind these preventable deaths were frequently embedded in the national culture and infrastructure. The SDGs did take an important step in their reframing of maternal mortality within an emphasis on health and well-being across one's lifespan (goal three includes access to sexual and reproductive health care and health education, among other items) (UN n.d.), but to expect countries to be able to shift gears and create holistic approaches to health and well-being was a lot to ask. The health targets in the SDGs encompassed a host of health-related issues, which each required complex interconnected responses from the health-care sector and beyond. As such, if countries like Mexico were to address the many concerns laid out in the SDGs, they would "need to take the health sector out of isolation with more focus on illness prevention and promotion of well-being, and more collaboration with other sectors that influence health and illness outcomes" (Buse and Hawkes 2015, 6).

For the midwives I worked with, as well as many doctors and policymakers who spoke at women's health events across Mexico, there was a clear awareness of the connections between health outcomes and social conditions. Indeed, this book is largely an exploration of the creative ways Mexican midwives tried to bring attention to—and build lasting responses to—the social conditions that they saw affecting their patients' health. In stepping back from initiatives like the individual targets of the MDGs or the SDGs, the bigger picture shows there *is* recognition for the need for multipronged interventions—the need to address everything all at once. But what seems to happen is the symptoms of social inequality are addressed while the root causes continue. Roots are much harder to change than what breaks through to the surface.

While there are certainly shared features of these social inequalities worldwide—similar legacies of colonialism, economic fractures, infrastructural breakdowns, racism, and violence—the patterns they take vary. It makes sense for the symptoms to be the target of global initiatives, because it is easier to compare education levels, HIV rates, or maternal deaths across sites than to come up with universally applicable solutions to situated conditions of inequality or poverty.

One proposed solution to the gap between global development goals and the underlying problems at local and national levels is to pay more attention to grassroots initiatives. These "locally led, globally supported, and politically smart approaches" make sense because they understand both the specific conditions of the region as well as the ways that their population stacks up to global development indicators (Buse and Hawkes 2015, 5). However, an investment in local approaches seems in many ways antithetical to the universalizing approach of global health. To gain and maintain relevance, midwives have had to build a case for the connection between the work they do on a local level, which reflects the changing needs and contexts of their communities, and the goals of global health, which privilege projects that can be replicated over time and space.

"What We Offer": Midwives and the Strategic Use of Maternal Mortality

When Diana described her push to incorporate gynecology and to teach her students at Mujeres Aliadas how to make up for failures in the health-care system, she was trying to walk this middle ground. She was, as I described in the Introduction, working with the state and global development goals in the sense that she was framing her intervention (midwifery education and care that included laboratory testing and holistic health care across the lifespan to marginalized populations) as one which could ultimately help Mexico achieve development goals (reduce maternal deaths). But she did so strategically, for infused in her plan was a critical stance against the state's approach to women and women's health care, and against the narrowly focused target of maternal mortality reduction. This approach of strategically talking about maternal mortality above all other potential health indicators as a way to gain political support was increasingly shared among the administrators of the different schools where I worked, and it was being explicitly passed down to the students as well (see Chapter 1 for a discussion of CASA students being taught to engage in political activism).

One winter afternoon, as I sat with Renata, Diana's administrative partner at the Mujeres Aliadas midwifery school, I asked her about the growing emphasis on maternal mortality. She explained that, for her, the emphasis was definitely strategic. It was a discussion tool that could bring midwifery to the table with policy makers who otherwise might not be open to considering the possible roles midwives could play in the health-care system. "That is just what we need to sell; it is what we offer," she told me. "We need to tell them [the policy makers] that we can reduce maternal mortality! We just need to incorporate professional midwives into the system." I asked her if she thought that the conversation around maternal mortality was an easier "sell" to policy makers than arguments about humanizing birth. She nodded and replied, "I think so. It has more impact, more interest. They have their goals." By this, she referred to the maternal mortality reduction targets being discussed at every level of government, especially in regions of Mexico where the levels were still far above what the county had promised to achieve through the MDGs. Renata argued that midwives needed to explicitly address those specific goals, to show clearly how midwifery could help the state meet them.

The issues that Mujeres Aliadas was trying to target through its holistic approach to women's health do not sound trivial: undiagnosed vaginal infections, faulty laboratory test results, mistreatment by medical facility staff, a lack of systematic care and follow up for women with cervical cancer. The problem is that these issues do not always rise to the level of concern to warrant systematic global intervention, but that is because they do not get noticed, noted, and analyzed. If Diana had not caught her patient's inconsistent lab results, the patient may not have gotten treatment for her cervical cancer. These things can just happen—women can simply not know, and the lack of quality care can simply be overlooked. It takes dying for a woman's lack of health care to be noticed, registered, and made to count on a global level.

Diana's concerns about gynecological health and the bigger pushback against the effects of decades of global health policies focusing on maternal mortality reduction are symptoms of bigger tensions in the world of global health: between universal goals and local realities and between measurable outcomes and all the daily needs that go unaccounted for because they are harder to count.

A problem with creating universal goals in health care is that the details of how people experience health and illness and how they access care is different across countries and contexts. Therefore, expecting all divergent paths—be they highways or dirt roads—to converge at the same place and time makes little sense. But what is the alternative? Biomedicine has done a good job of spreading its institutions, technologies, and tools worldwide, and there has followed the notion that with such successful spread comes the possibility of universal health. But when lab tests have conflicting results, when there are shortages of medicines or medical tools, or when practitioners act on biomedical authority in performing outdated or dangerous practices (see Chapter 4), we get further from the universal goal. Supporting grassroots, local initiatives that better understand the actual needs and expectations of the people, as well as the actual availability of resources at hand, makes sense if we want to address underlying factors leading to poor health outcomes.

It is important to note that the emphasis on maternal mortality reduction as the central focus of women's health during the past few decades is not the first or only way that women's reproductive processes and possibilities have been targeted as development indicators. Indeed, women's choices around whether, when, and how to have children have long been of interest to the state, as evidenced through Mexican fertility control campaigns that aimed to "promote economic development in the southern hemisphere through disarming the 'population bomb' by lowering birth rates around the globe" (Gutmann 2011, 54). I had seen how such campaigns could make women feel like their fertility was the only thing about their bodies worth discussing. In 2004, years before beginning my doctoral program and the research that makes up this book, I was living in Oaxaca City in southern Mexico and continuing to learn about midwifery. My day job, however, was as a qualitative researcher for a Mexican NGO called the Mexican Institute for Family and Population (IMIFAP), which focused on health, education, and community development. IMIFAP was conducting a cervical cancer prevention project that was trying to gauge rural women's understanding of sexual and reproductive health and determine best practices for cervical cancer education, prevention, and treatment.[3] My role, along with a team of other trained researchers, was to conduct door-to-door interviews about sexual and reproductive health with hundreds of women in rural outlying villages to gauge their knowledge level, then return to interview their neighbors after a team of *promotoras* (lay health promoters) had led the villages in trainings about cervical cancer. We were hoping to show that the trainings had worked and that the information had spread, though the results were rather mixed in the end. As part of the project, I also assisted a team of providers in conducting free pap smear clinics in every town where we were working.

Having already conducted hundreds of interviews with this population, I was not surprised that most of the women we saw had not only never had a pap smear but also had rarely been to a doctor except possibly for pregnancy and childbirth. These were private women, for whom talking about sexual health and their bodies did not come easily—especially with a stranger (and a foreigner, at that).

I was interviewing a woman in her home, and I asked her what I thought (and what had seemed in prior interviews) to be a simple introductory question, listed in the demographic questions that preceded the tougher questions about sexuality and sexual health: "How many children do you have, *señora?*" Instead of answering automatically, like all the others had done before her, she suddenly looked sad. "I have four," she said then quickly added, "but I felt bad about that." I was confused—she felt bad about having four children? I asked her what she meant, and she explained that, when the youngest was a baby, they had to take him to Mexico City to see a specialist for some health issues. The doctor there asked her how many children she had, and when she told him that she had four, he scolded her. "He told me that 2.5 was the correct number of children we should be having in Mexico," she said to me. "How can you have 2.5 children?" I asked her, aghast. "Well, he explained that it was an average, but he still made me feel bad for having more than the correct number." What does it mean for women to be told they have "too many" children? In this case, the doctor was passing along the idea of national targets for fertility to his patient in a way that made her ashamed of her own reproductive history even years later as she recounted the story to me.

Anthropologists have increasingly been documenting the effects of the global fascination with the universalizing promise of metrics as a tool and product of globalization (Adams 2016), especially as they become translated into clinical encounters like the one above. In the realm of women's health, these metrics have focused increasingly on maternal mortality rates. As Nicole Berry points out, even as maternal mortality stands as an insufficient marker for the health and social issues women are most concerned about, the ways it is being studied are inadequate; as she says, "We neglect the myriad rich and important other sources of data that might help us mitigate some of these deaths" (2010, 2). For the midwives, infrastructural and obstetric violence (discussed in Chapters 3 and 4) were the real culprits of maternal deaths.

While global health initiatives such as the push to reduce maternal mortality can and do further alienate traditionally marginalized practitioners like midwives, the midwives I worked with were also trying to use these initiatives to hold their ground. The complex negotiations between global health campaigns and local practitioners are not, of course, limited to Mexico: Berry found that, in Guatemala, global campaigns to reduce maternal mortality allowed health-care workers who already saw traditional practitioners like midwives as "backward" to justify their prejudice toward them within "an objective, neutral framework" (2010, 4). What stood out to me in Mexico was how the midwives were able to put their own, self-serving spin on these campaigns. "Hire us," they were saying, "and we can not only reduce maternal mortality, but we can improve women's experiences and reduce costs, as well."

In her analysis of midwifery and maternal health in Mexico, Williams lays bare what the midwives were doing as they appealed to the state and global health communities with their promises of maternal mortality reduction and their critiques of how the state had bungled its attempts thus far. She says that

> midwives and midwifery advocates explicitly connect Mexico's failure to meet its maternal health MDGs and reduce its MMR to the high rates of obstetric violence in the country, arguing that obstetric violence isn't a side project to be addressed after MMR is improved but is, rather, key to improving not only MMR but also the affective experiences of women during birth. Midwives also read MMR as an indictment of the failed project of overmedicalization during childbirth, and leverage Mexico's stalled rate in support of their own push for midwifery to be recognized and incorporated into the public health system. (2019, 8)

I agree that midwives were leveraging Mexico's maternal mortality concerns to advocate for their own approach to care, but I do not necessarily see this as something about which to be critical. Rather, I see their efforts as opportunistic and strategic; they were finding ways to link their ongoing concerns about infrastructure and the treatment of women in Mexico to concerns that had garnered more attention. In this way, the midwives tied their experiences with individual women and communities to state interests that were motivated by larger global initiatives. It is not only the midwives being strategic, of course. Given the historical linkages between the Mexican government, global trends, and modernization projects, when state officials announce their support for global policies (such as maternal mortality reduction), their motivations are not always clear; indeed, it may not be possible to tease apart international pressures, national modernization ideals, and grassroots influences (Dion 2008). In working both with and against the health-care system on the issue of maternal mortality, midwives were trying to force local, state, national, and ultimately global campaigns to pay attention to issues that existed beyond, beneath, and because of maternal mortality. Issues like Mujeres Aliadas' patients' undetected cervical cancer or chronic vaginal infections, or the lack of hospital beds and poor treatment of women described in the chapters that follow.

Conclusion

The midwives I worked with were arguing, on the one hand, that the system was deeply broken and that they should be employed by the state to fill in the gaps—gaps through which they saw their patients slipping. They were using global campaigns, and especially the emphasis on maternal mortality reduction, to justify the need for their profession. Midwives, they argued, are affordable, flexible, and accepted by their communities, ideal qualifications to bring care to populations whom the state cannot always access. Yet the midwives were also saying that the system would not be fixed any time soon, and they could offer a more long-term solution in a context where universal access to resources and standardized quality control of services were far from being achieved.

I was talking to the owner of a medical testing facility in central Mexico recently, and I shared with her the story of the patient with the conflicting lab results. "Oh yeah," she said, nodding as I spoke. "This happens all the time—that is why I started sending out our samples for independent verification." She explained that her facility always double tests their samples. "I just don't understand how this woman's test results could be so different," I said, still grappling with the potentially devastating consequences of missing a cancer diagnosis. "You should see some of these . . . 'labs,'" she said, forming air quotes with her fingers. "They are just someone's kitchen with some test tubes set up. It is criminal." She mentioned the lack of oversight, the state not having the time or resources to control all the testing facilities. I thought again about Mujeres Aliadas; by teaching her students to do their own lab tests, Diane was rendering the services they had to offer more appealing to the state (because it was one less thing for the state to have to do), while simultaneously improving their patients' quality of care.

Midwives had learned the hard way that they had to do a sort of dance for the Mexican state. They had to perform their expertise in a way that biomedical practitioners did not, because their expertise was taken for granted as system insiders. The midwives had to learn the language of global health and development and artfully insert themselves into a narrative that long vilified them: whereas midwives used to be seen as antithetical to the goals of global development, these midwives argued that they offered a surprising solution.

Not all the midwives I talked to felt great about this dance. Some felt strongly that they should not have to justify their profession to doctors, to the health secretary, to the world; they felt that they were giving their patients and communities what they wanted and thus should be allowed to continue to practice on those merits alone. Yet overwhelmingly, the message I received was that midwives had to be strategic and political. They had to keep up with the messaging around what counts in global health and continue to find ways to make themselves appear indispensable. They had to be made to matter, even if—as many of them saw it—the women they cared for did not always appear to matter very much to the state. As one midwifery school administrator put it, bluntly, during a meeting with state representatives, "Mexico doesn't actually care about women." She meant that government policies were not made with women's desires or experiences in mind. Midwives learned that the quickest way to help the women they cared for was not to try to convince politicians otherwise; rather, they would help women by making midwifery a valid and state-sanctioned option, thus giving women the opportunity to choose a different kind of health care, one which could address their health needs beyond the moment of reproduction.

There are critiques of the midwives' implied connection between support of midwives and improved health outcomes for Mexico. Whether midwives can make enough of an impact in Mexico to really chip away at the maternal mortality ratio is a little murky; there just are not that many midwives in practice. Further, it is not easy to show how humanized birth and holistic health care lead to reductions in maternal mortality, as midwives argue. Yet it is also hard to mount counter arguments against what midwives are saying: that the system is broken and that supporting midwives might be a way to start filling in some of its gaps and perhaps, ultimately, improve health outcomes.

When midwives talked about the system being "broken," they did so from a unique perspective. Many midwives, like those training at Mujeres Aliadas, worked inside the health-care system. They encountered its systemic failures on a daily basis and saw how such failures affected women. Yet in training to become midwives, they were learning how to be critical of the systems in which they worked, to see the failures as more than just material but rather as both products of and productive of structural inequalities that shaped women's health experiences and outcomes. The effects of such inequalities are not unique to Mexico. As countries across the world—including the United States—grapple with the persistence of preventable maternal deaths, it has become clear that there is not a simple fix. Centuries of social inequality, structural violence, racism, and discrimination play out tragically in delivery rooms and bedrooms across the developed as well as the developing world: when women do not have adequate support and care throughout their pregnancy, birth, and postpartum period, they are at risk. The next chapter looks more closely at these structural inequalities and the conditions they create for women and asks: given these conditions, where might midwives intervene, and can they effect real change from inside a broken system?

CHAPTER 3

Maternal Conditions

Irma's Story

On October 2, 2013, Irma López Aurelio—a pregnant, Indigenous woman of Mazateco origins—arrived at the local hospital in the southern Mexican state of Oaxaca to have her baby. As her labor progressed over the next two hours, she tried repeatedly to get help from the staff but was ignored. Eventually she made her way to the patio of the hospital and gave birth, unassisted, in the grass. It was there that Irma was captured on film in a photograph that soon went viral across Mexican news media sources. In the photograph, Irma bears a frantic expression as she half kneels on the ground holding up the hem of her dress. Her baby, crying and still connected to her by the umbilical cord, lies on the grass beneath her.

What journalists were quick to point out was that Irma's case was not rare. Public outcry reached all the way to the Mexican national secretary of health, and statements were made about the efforts of the Mexican government to increase emergency obstetric training among its health-care workers (*La prensa* 2013). Irma's story tells one part of a larger narrative about the pervasive inequalities that direct the kinds of reproductive health care women are receiving today in Mexico. But even for those women who have gained access to care during pregnancy and delivery, another realm of injustice still exists—including the use of forced sterilizations and lack of informed consent procedures, the archaic and unnecessary manual removal of placentas,[1] the overuse of cesarean sections and episiotomies (INEGI 2015; Jesús-García et al. 2018), and the outright mistreatment of women in labor (Zacher Dixon 2015; Smith-Oka 2015). And then there are those women who do not even have nearby access to care or find that the care to which they do have access is not what they had hoped—as in Irma's case.

The fact that Irma was from a poor, rural, Indigenous community did not escape the attention of the press. Indeed, underneath the photograph of her birth the magazine cover read: "Mazatec begged for two hours for them to attend her: Hospital in Oaxaca forces Indigenous woman to give birth on the grass" (Coatecatl 2013, my translation). The headline doubly emphasizes her identity as part of a marginalized group: first by naming her as Mazatec, referencing the people who live in the Sierra Mazateca of Oaxaca and neighboring states, and second by calling her an Indigenous woman. Her experience of the Mexican health-care system cannot be separated from who she is. In a country where dramatic divides between rich and poor, light skinned and dark skinned, urban and rural determine access and treatment in the medical system and beyond, Irma fell squarely into the category of lowest priority, a category in which she was not alone. Studies have shown that women in Mexico, as elsewhere, who have lower socioeconomic status, get pregnant younger, live in marginalized rural areas further from metropolitan centers, and have lower education levels are more likely to have less prenatal care than women without these barriers (Heredia-Pi et al. 2016). While maternal mortality ratios have decreased in Mexico overall, and access to care for pregnant women has increased in much of the country, historically marginalized regions like Irma's state of Oaxaca (alongside Chiapas and Guerrero) continue to lag behind more prosperous, less historically marginalized, Indigenous states (Rodríguez-Aguilar 2018). Irma was born into a hierarchical society shaped by colonialism, racism, and classism, and her own birth story could be read as her physical embodiment of those legacies (Krieger 2005). Looked at from another angle, an analysis of her birth tells us a lot about how she lived. Indeed, as childbirth educator Gayle Peterson once said, "As a woman lives, so shall she give birth, so shall she die" (1984, 3). What in Irma's history and identity led her to give birth in this way?

As childbirth experiences and outcomes worldwide have come under increased scrutiny, Peterson's quote continues to ring true. In both developed and developing countries, women's social status is a major determining factor for their health in pregnancy and birth. In the United States, for example, maternal mortality is actually on the *rise* (MacDorman et al. 2016). We are beginning to understand the links between gender inequality, social violence, access to education and reproductive health care, and maternal health outcomes (Hunt, Bueno, and Mesquita 2007). If we want to help women, then we need to address these underlying issues.

In Mexico, as elsewhere, women's experiences and outcomes in pregnancy and birth come to stand in for the legacies of racism and inequality that continue to shape daily life. Irma's birth should shock and surprise us in its brutality and irony—she got herself to a clinic, followed the rules, and still ended up abandoned by the system—yet it does not; Irma was indeed one of the lucky ones. She and her baby were both deemed healthy in the end.[2] Many other women across Mexico, especially women like Irma—poor, Indigenous, rural women—do not survive pregnancy or labor.

As in Irma's case, how women give birth can tell us a lot about what is going on in their communities and countries, how priorities in health-care initiatives have been designed, and how health outcomes map onto existing patterns of social inequality. Reproductive politics—and the politics of childbirth in particular—reflect changing beliefs about women's agency and the state's responsibility regarding care. In Mexico, the United Nations' Millennium Development Goals and their central emphasis on reduced maternal mortality as the primary indicator of a good outcome have largely defined the past two decades of women's health initiatives (as described in Chapter 2). While the reduction in maternal mortality was universally accepted as a noble goal, the way that it has shaped interventions in Mexico has led many to question the potential dangers of its centrality. In turn, such questions reflect pressing concerns about the mismatch between what counts as progress and how situations like Irma's could happen despite the purported great strides in development and modernization in countries like Mexico (Cortés 2013).

In this chapter, I look at how infrastructural inequalities in Mexico have contributed to the widening of fissures between those who have access to safe, respectful reproductive health care and those who do not. I describe what I call "maternal conditioning": a term I use to refer both to the process through which women *become conditioned* to behaving in a certain way and expecting certain things and to the material *conditions* that women find themselves in once they act as they are told. As a process, maternal conditioning is what happens to make women do what the state needs them to do. As an outcome, maternal conditions are not ideal for many women in Mexico, as across the world. Beneath these two things—the process and the outcome—lies the history of national efforts to shift Mexico from a developing country to a developed one by, in part, making sure women don't die in childbirth. In the previous chapter, I discussed the process through which global development policies aimed at reducing maternal mortality affect women's health outcomes and experiences in sometimes unexpected ways. This chapter, however, looks more specifically at the infrastructures that both reveal and reproduce unequal conditions for many women across Mexico, like Irma.

This chapter is, at its core, about patient-provider interactions and the factors that shape them. As such, I add to a wealth of scholarship that has brought to light the relationships among socio-historical context, infrastructure, and health care, within the broader Mexican health-care context and in the field of reproductive health more generally. Whitney Duncan (2017) and Beatriz Reyes-Foster (2018), for example, show how mental health practitioners and their patients in Mexico struggle toward a modern vision of health while simultaneously confronting the limiting realities of living the effects of colonialism, economic insecurity, and marginalization. Lucia Guerra-Reyes's (2019) work on birth in the Peruvian Andes reveals how even seemingly inclusive maternal health policies, like Peru's Intercultural Birthing Policy, cannot break entrenched infrastructures built to curtail women's choices in health care. The structures that shape women's choices and experiences are not always physical, of course; Dána-Ain Davis's (2019) work brings to light the ways that Black women and babies' health outcomes in the United States continue to be affected by the legacy of slavery and the persistence of racism throughout the health-care system. Here, I posit that reproductive health-care infrastructures cannot be separated from such socio-historical legacies but rather are tightly linked to them.

But how do we make visible these linkages? Below, I discuss the concept of "infrastructural violence" to illustrate the ways that unequal care can be mapped onto entrenched inequalities within built environments, institutional legacies, and inherited practices. I describe how such seemingly disparate problems—such as a lack of radio repeater towers, national programs for staffing rural clinics, or poor road conditions—cumulatively represent the uneven ways that resources, knowledge, and access are distributed throughout developing countries. I then describe some of the ways that midwives are trying to address this infrastructural violence through a humanization of the health-care system. As such, I show how they are casting themselves as indispensable to Mexico because of their ability to bridge infrastructural gaps, to mend failings in the system, and to address issues of resource scarcity, knowledge deficiencies, and lack of access—all without too hefty a price tag. If the midwives are able to patch themselves into this infrastructure, they argue, they may be able to build a sustainable future for their profession while bringing better care to the women who need it the most.

What Is the Infrastructure?

The Mexican health-care system has changed considerably in the past twenty years, and it continues to change under the new Andrés Manuel López Obrador presidency. Many of the changes have been made in the name of extending state services to marginalized populations. The Mexican health-care system is basically divided into two main segments—private and public. About a quarter of the population relies on privately purchased insurance or just direct payments to providers, though this segment makes up about half of Mexico's total health expenditure (Doubova et al., "Barriers," 2018, 1074). The other 75 percent of the population relies on public insurance programs, which make up the other half of Mexico's total health expenditure. Those with jobs in the formal labor market are associated with programs under the Mexican Institute of Social Security,[3] while those who do not have formal jobs that pay into such programs qualify for Seguro Popular (Popular Health Insurance) (Doubova et al., "Barriers," 2018). The creation of Seguro Popular in 2003 was a response to the high numbers of people who were not covered by any health-insurance program and provided free or low-cost services to a large segment of the population. It has indeed increased access to care for a large part of the population. With Seguro Popular came the message that health care was a universal right that the government recognized for its people (R. Castro 2014).

However, the realities behind the numbers show that despite admirable increases in access to care, many Mexicans continue to fall through the cracks. One explanation is the fragmentation of the current health-care system, in which patients may not receive continuity of care across different types of insurance or institutions, or the quality of care may vary considerably depending on where they go (Doubova et al., "Barriers," 2018). Another explanation has been that, while reports have shown that most Mexican people now have some kind of insurance coverage, detailed analysis reveals that the numbers may be masking the reality: on the one hand, many people have multiple kinds of insurance (private insurance and ISSSTE, for example), which makes it seem like more people have insurance than actually do, and on the other hand, just having Seguro Popular does not guarantee access—many rural areas are without services or are understaffed (R. Castro 2014; Gómez Dantés et al. 2011). Indeed, a recent study showed that, despite the expansion of Seguro Popular, those who can pay for private care are still at a great advantage, as "half of available examining rooms and hospital beds in the country are private" (Doubova et al., "Quality," 2018, e1149).

Despite this uneven coverage, the rhetoric has largely been that, with the option of Seguro Popular, nobody needs to go to a care provider who exists outside formal systems, such as midwives. In this way, the idea that Mexican people have a right to health care also comes with a heavily implied responsibility—the responsibility to use the health care being provided by the state, even if it is far away, it does not offer evidence-based, quality care, or you prefer to see a midwife instead. Women are conditioned to believe that they have to get to a state clinic or hospital for their care, no matter what—even if the conditions they find there are less than ideal. Smith-Oka (2013) describes how this conditioning leads women to feel the need to express deep gratitude toward doctors and health-care institutions, even if they have experienced painful, scary, or bad care and even if the providers have treated them with open prejudice. Patients admitted to Smith-Oka how terrible their experiences in birth actually were, but they felt the need to perform the role of the "good patient" by appearing thankful.

One doctor working in an overcrowded Seguro Popular labor ward told me how he had conflicting views about the increasing use of these hospitals by the population. "Before Seguro Popular," he explained, "people would save their money to pay for a delivery. Now, even those who could pay to go to a less crowded, private hospital for care are choosing to spend that money on something else and come here for free instead." The doctor understood that the financial incentive helped a lot of women and families, but he also felt that those who could pay to go elsewhere were taking up beds needed by the poorest of the population and creating a situation of overcrowding that perpetuated poor quality of care.

Infrastructural Violence and Maternal Conditioning

Programs like Seguro Popular provided important services for many; for pregnant women, Seguro Popular meant that they had a place to go for emergencies (cesareans, preterm labor, hemorrhage, or any of the other potentially life-threatening issues that can arise in pregnancy and postpartum). Indeed, midwives agreed that state facilities such as those run by Seguro Popular were necessary to attending women with high-risk deliveries or complications—nobody argued that all women should birth outside hospitals. Rather, midwives argued that women should have the choice of with whom they wanted to deliver, and that wherever they sought care, they should receive humane, dignified treatment. Yet midwives saw broken infrastructures and the mistreatment of women as systemic conditions that many of them argued could lead to poor outcomes. When women are conditioned to seek biomedical care for reproductive health, they confront both of these issues and find themselves in conditions that make it hard for them to have good outcomes or positive experiences. For the midwives I worked with, these conditions presented obvious problems that clearly stood in the way of achieving the very goals that they shared with the state—to reduce maternal death. Many of the midwives felt frustrated that the very conditions developed to help women had become the poor conditions that hurt them.

The impacts on the health-care infrastructure of prioritizing maternal mortality reduction through medicalizing childbirth have been far reaching and often result in such jarring cases and public outcry as that which arose from Irma's case. Many of the midwives, doctors, and activists I spoke with asked: How can we push women to give birth in hospitals, but then not offer them safe passage or a bed in which to give birth when they arrive? What happens if we remove women's safety nets—their local practitioners—without first ensuring that they will be cared for? These questions were especially important for those working and living in rural, remote communities where access to the kinds of hospitals where women were urged to go was often much more difficult. Uneven access to state health-care facilities, poor road conditions, lack of radio or cellular communication, and inconsistent emergency transportation all contributed to uneven infrastructures that could make it harder for some women to get care; resource scarcity, lack of beds or medications, and understaffed clinics or hospitals all made it hard to get good care once the women got to a facility.

Taken together, these conditions, coupled with the state's emphasis on clinic or hospital births, represent a type of "infrastructural violence" (Rodgers and O'Neill 2012) that women—particularly those living in rural regions—face when trying to access quality reproductive health care. Infrastructures matter on many registers. While the concept of infrastructure was long ignored by anthropologists because it seemed uninteresting and apolitical, Susan Leigh Star (1999) brought attention to the many ways that infrastructure indeed reveals power dynamics, social conventions, and complex relationships, both in its construction and in its breakdown. Indeed, Marco Di Nunzio points out that infrastructure is assumed to be about serving the public good, but that "as ethnographers and geographers have pointed out, building infrastructure is not a neutral endeavor. While continuing to embody visions of progress, pipelines, highways, and electric lines serve vested interests, enforce regimes of control, and create geographies of abjection and segregation" (2018, 1). I use the term "infrastructure" here to refer to the physical structures, built world, and health-care system organization that collectively reinforce social inequalities by privileging the few and marginalizing many. Infrastructure appears blameless in its inhuman form, but, the midwives argue through their reclamations of infrastructural failings and the politics behind them, it is indeed both human and inhumane: it is built by humans, and it inhumanely creates the conditions in which many women are set up to fail.

The concept of infrastructural violence builds on Paul Farmer's (2004) definition of structural violence, but it refers specifically to the material channels through which structural violence flows (Rodgers and O'Neill 2012). Rodgers and O'Neill helpfully distinguish between active infrastructural violence (things planned and built with an intention to survey, divide, or restrict access, such as low bridges that do not allow public buses into certain spaces or streets designed to provide security to a city) and passive infrastructural violence (which references the limitations or omissions of infrastructure). Both of these variations operate to shape the maternal health landscape across Mexico. Certain spaces like labor and delivery wards are designed in ways that may constitute active infrastructural violence (in that they do not allow space for women to have partners present during birth, for example), while other attributes of infrastructure (such as poor roads, a lack of local schools, overcrowded health centers, or a lack of radio repeater towers) allow for violence to happen passively, by structuring the possibilities for neglect, especially in rural regions. When certain bodies are unable to access infrastructures, the suffering that they experience and which marks their bodies and communities (as in when maternal mortality rates are higher in rural regions where there are no good routes to emergency medical services) "only serves to facilitate forms of social exclusion that fundamentally question notions of citizenship, rights, and membership claims by the poor and otherwise vulnerable" (Rodgers and O'Neill 2012, 407).

While infrastructural violence affects marginalized groups across Mexico, its impact on women in rural regions is significant. As described in Chapter 1, the rural–urban divisions that persist in statistics about Mexican health outcomes and education levels are deeply linked to legacies of colonialism and racism. Karen Rignall posits that rurality is in some forms itself a kind of gender violence, in that it "grows out of historically-situated and material practices that have rendered aspects of rural life disproportionately dangerous or difficult for women" (2019, 19). In her case, Rignall is trying to show how women experience structural violence in rural regions of Morocco differently than men do, not (only) because of ideas of tradition or Islamic patriarchy that constrain them but because of systemic power forces (of which, she argues, patriarchy is only one branch). Similarly, I found that in Mexico, ideas of tradition, machismo, and conservative Catholicism are often proposed to explain women's reproductive choices and outcomes, when again, these are only one part of the power dynamic that leads to women's unequal access to health care and health outcomes. Blaming culture for women's inability to get to a clinic in time or even to survive childbirth is an updated version of the nineteenth-century narrative about the rural Indigenous population, who were charged as somehow at fault for their own misery (instead of being recognized as victims of horrible, inhumane working conditions, for example) (Soto Laveaga 2013).

When already marginalized women are conditioned to seek out biomedical care in a setting where getting that care can be impossible, by being told by health workers that they must have their babies in clinics or hospitals, even when those are hours away, overcrowded, or provide low-quality care, they are experiencing the paradoxical effects of infrastructural violence: because infrastructures are assumed to be for the public good, those who do not use them appear to be lazy, uneducated, or out of control. To call this paradox out as violence forces us to pay attention to the ways that roads and radios, ambulances and beds can all be markers of privilege; those who do not have them suffer violently in their absence.

The failings in Mexico's health infrastructure are not hard to see, and my point is not that I am uncovering some hidden breakdown. This was a common topic of popular discussion during my research, one that midwives and politicians alike returned to again and again when discussing the never-ending list of things that needed improving. What I point out is that in the face of the scale of these failings, when there is so much to be done to fully extend the infrastructure to all (if this is even a possibility), midwifery continues to make sense as a profession that can, to some degree, close the gap. Midwives may not be able to build the roads or restock the clinics, but they can bring good care to those who cannot get to good care otherwise, and that is a start.

In 2012, I attended a national meeting of midwives, policy makers, researchers, and doctors who were all interested in addressing problems with the ways women were being treated during childbirth in Mexican public hospitals. Martina, a researcher from Fundar research center in Mexico City, presented on this issue at the conference.

Mexico, she said, has only .63 beds per 1,000 people who don't have health insurance or depend on Seguro Popular, which is far below the WHO's recommended one bed per 1,000 people. In marginalized places, she said, this statistic is even worse—dropping to .1 beds per 1,000 people. Such statistics, she pointed out, made clearer the alarming finding that around a third of the maternal deaths registered in recent years were women who had Seguro Popular. For Martina, then, having access to Seguro Popular did not mean that women were being seen or attended to, especially if there were not even enough beds for patients.

Doctors reiterated her argument during the conference, citing times when they had seen women waiting outside in long lines to be seen at the Seguro Popular hospital, even when in active labor (a scene which reflects the frequency of experiences like Irma's). Dr. Ramirez, an obstetrician from Oaxaca who advocated for systemic changes to Mexico's maternal health infrastructure, said that the country is in a "profound crisis" with regards to low-risk births. He explained that, under programs like Seguro Popular, women are compelled to go to bigger hospitals for their births even if they are in low-risk categories and could have given birth at least in their local clinics with general practitioners or even professional midwives. These low-risk births are, he argued, clogging up the system for those who have high-risk situations and need the care of a bigger hospital.

Renata, the administrator at Mujeres Aliadas midwifery school, repeated this point during an interview some months later. "Maternal mortality is *rising* in hospitals!" she told me. "It is because of oversaturation. Social programs like Seguro Popular grew too quickly, and they couldn't keep up. They can't! How are they going to offer services to the whole population when they don't have the infrastructure?" Both Renata and Dr. Ramirez's concerns echoed what I heard midwives discuss regularly; there were frequently just not enough beds, and sometimes it could be hard to know if the women who needed level one hospital attention (in the larger, more equipped hospitals located in bigger cities) were the ones who were getting the beds.

This situation was brought into sharp focus for me one day in San Miguel de Allende as I chatted with a woman in town after I had left CASA for the day. She had asked me what my research was about and, when I told her, she laughed and said lightly that she herself had a fine birth at the local hospital and probably would not have ever considered a midwife. I asked what her experience was like, and she paused then said that she thought it had felt like "a competition," because there were so many women lined up in the crowded labor room, each trying to get through labor alone (they were not allowed anyone with them because of the high volume of patients and privacy concerns). While this woman found this crowded environment stimulating, other women I spoke to did not. Indeed, many women who came to CASA for prenatal care shared that they did not want to repeat such conditions as they had endured during previous births at the large public hospitals.

One solution for dealing with overcrowding in these urban hospitals was to disperse patients to regional clinics. Many smaller cities and towns already had health centers that could attend lower-risk births, and many midwives, policy-makers, and activists argued that midwives should also be able to attend low-risk pregnancies, especially when even these health centers were too far away.

Some people I talked to raised concerns about sending women to give birth at local health centers, arguing that even when they existed with the purpose of providing local care for Mexico's more rural regions, they did not provide a consistent level of care. Dr. Garza (a general practice doctor who helped train CASA midwives) lamented to me that these rural clinics were tricky because the providers were fresh out of medical school, without any specialized training and with little hands-on experience. In Mexico, Dr. Garza explained, most doctors never sought out a specialization, creating a situation that looked much the opposite of the United States—in Mexico, most doctors are general practitioners, and only a few are specialists, while in the United States, current concerns about primary care shortages (Dall 2018) are seen as the result of decades of pushing doctors to specialize. Dr. Garza saw specializing as something that was difficult for many of his peers—it required more money and time, and, he told me, the need to read English (the language of much of the materials and journals one needs to read to stay up to date within a specialization). Most doctors in Mexico did not go on to complete a specialization, then, but were still tasked with a wide range of practice in their jobs—especially if they were the only provider posted in a small, rural town.

These rural health centers were staffed through Mexico's system of enforced service for many medical professionals; after completing medical school, young doctors were sent to a clinic for a year. This system, begun under President Lázaro Cárdenas in the 1930s (Mills 2010), both helped new practitioners gain practice and confidence and kept the health centers staffed; it was also necessary in part because many practitioners would not voluntarily choose to live and work in rural regions of Mexico, so this was a way to ensure there was some level of care there. CASA founder Nadine argued, however, that it was not a perfect system—in fact, she saw it as another symptom of an unequal system. "It is basically the best example of racism you can get," she said, "when the rural people of Mexico are being treated like guinea pigs for doctors just coming out of school where they did not have hands-on, supervised training." Indeed, when the requirement for this social service was rolled out in 1936, it was framed as "one of the most singular experiments that has ever been recorded in the history of medicine" (González 1981, 280; my translation). This forced medical social service has also been analyzed as a tool of post-revolutionary control, which not only taught urban practitioners to treat rural patients but also brought state surveillance into rural regions; in addition, the practitioners were there to teach the masses what kind of medical knowledge counted and who could officially practice it. At the same time, those practitioners sent home depictions of rural populations that reinforced stereotypes of them as lazy or alcoholic (Soto Laveaga 2013). While not everyone I spoke to agreed with Nadine's assessment of these rural clinics as experimental and therefore potentially unethical, many did worry that the local resources were not enough to address women's reproductive health needs. Indeed, Mexico's National Commission on Human Rights has received numerous complaints about the lack of supervision that these newly minted doctors receive (Mills 2010).

Dr. Jones, a physician who worked in Mexico coordinating trainings in emergency obstetrics, raised a similar concern when I interviewed him. He noted, "If you asked a typical intern in the US if they would be ready to go practice right now, they'd be like, 'no! I'm not ready!'" Dr. Jones's trainings sought to bring much-needed information to medical students who might be faced with obstetric complications after never having dealt with them in school. Part of that work involved re-training practicing physicians in the best practices in obstetric emergencies, since many of them had never really received advanced training in that area, despite years of work delivering babies. One example Dr. Jones brought up, which was reiterated by other doctors throughout my fieldwork, was many physicians' reluctance to use magnesium sulfate to treat preeclampsia and eclampsia, two major causes of maternal death in Mexico. Despite being very effective and cheap as a treatment, "everyone was terrified to use it, so they weren't using it," he explained. He went on to describe how his group went on to lead a workshop teaching the correct way to use the medication and dispelling concerns about its safety. Dr. Jones's trainings also emphasized the need for local practitioners (including midwives), emergency responders, and hospital personnel to work together and have a common language and set of practices to employ in cases of obstetric emergency, especially considering that it is not always feasible or safe to try to transfer women to the first-level hospitals when emergencies arise. He said that "probably 85 percent of the problems [in obstetrical care] could be resolved on the spot if they [the providers] knew what they were doing. But the typical reaction is 'get them out of here,' and then they die on the way." He said that when designing and implementing these trainings, attention to context was key—"We are always thinking about the context the provider is in." As he described it, the context sounded like one in which practitioners were not getting enough training to begin with and then were being sent out into areas where they had little mentorship, support, or recourse in cases of emergency. While Dr. Jones's work was making an impact, it did not address the infrastructural issues that necessitated his efforts in the first place.

The landscape of unequal care across Mexico, and especially across its rural regions, is not new. In 1938, Mexican anthropologist Miguel Othón de Mendizábal spoke about the vast disparities in care across his county at the Congress on Rural Medicine; nearly 70 percent of Mexican municipalities lacked a physician at that time, and these were primarily concentrated in states with higher Indigenous populations (Oaxaca, Puebla, Chiapas, Tlaxcala, México, Veracruz, and Yucatán) (Soto Laveaga 2013, 404). These regions continue to face shortages of providers, infrastructure, and resources for care. However, as Gabriela Soto Laveaga (2013) points out, the emphasis on increasing providers in rural regions (which, she notes, was also needed) deflected attention from the deeper issue leading to higher mortality rates among the rural poor: poverty.

For many of the midwives I spoke with, social inequality underlies the infrastructural violence that makes rural, Indigenous women more likely to die in childbirth. As one midwife lamented during a meeting with her fellow CASA graduates, "If the government really cared about rural women's health, they would make sure all the health providers—maybe even all the pregnant women—at least had radios." She explained that, in the rural regions where she was working in Guerrero, there was rarely cellular service and, without radios, providers could not get help for women in emergency situations. When I later asked a doctor about this situation, he agreed—but said that the problem went beyond handing out radios. First, you would need to even build the radio repeater towers, he told me. He went on to say, almost as an afterthought, that even if you could get through on a radio, sometimes the roads were so bad that help would arrive too late anyway, if it could arrive at all.

Bridging the Divide

A significant casualty of this infrastructural breakdown was the lack of trust many people felt toward the government, including state health services. Decades of experiences with crumbling roads, unequal levels of care, and unmet promises made by governments whose alliances shifted with changes in leadership every few years left many feeling disillusioned.

Over the years, as I followed midwives and their students into consult rooms and patients' living rooms, listening to them talk to patients and hearing the patients' concerns, I began to see how their trust in the health-care system had been eroded. Even though it was invisible, this lack of trust could stop women from getting good care just as tangibly as an eroded road or a lack of beds at a nearby clinic could. It was through decades of marginalization, shifting state messages about the Indigenous poor, and policies that did not always have women's best interest at heart that many women had come to feel that they should not engage with state agencies unless they absolutely had to. This resulted in women not always getting the treatment or oversight they needed and exacerbated the problems that could lead to complications later on (such as during pregnancy). The midwives were well aware of this trust issue, and a large part of their work seemed to involve attempts to overcome it. One important way that they tried to do this was by reaching out to women on the women's own terms, thus trying to bridge the divide between patient and provider and to remove any potential hurdles for getting care.

One autumn day I arrived early at the CASA clinic to attend a day of home visits with two students who had been assigned to follow up on patients they had seen throughout their pregnancies and births. The students—Alma (in her third and final year) and Yolanda (in her first year)—were waiting for me, and we all dug into the bag of warm empanadas I had picked up on the way as we headed immediately out to the bus stop. We were on our way to visit Rosa, a patient who had recently missed a postpartum visit at CASA and about whom one of the staff midwives was concerned. Rosa's water had broken early in her labor, and the midwife had been worried about an infection; she needed the students to assure her that Rosa remained symptom free a week out from labor.

"Does Rosa know we are coming today?" I asked Alma. I asked because the previous week I had tried to tag along during home visits, only to watch as the students tried and failed to reach patient after patient by phone before going to their homes. That day, the students had explained to me that many women simply do not want to be found or contacted. "They don't always trust us, they give us false numbers or addresses—sometimes we go there, and there isn't even a house there," they told me. I was initially shocked and confused by this, but the students explained that many of their patients were very wary of health-care providers because they had had negative experiences in the past. They did not understand why the midwives or their students would want to come to their homes, and so they were often evasive.

This day, however, Alma assured me that she had spoken with Rosa's mother before I arrived at CASA and had been told that someone would be waiting for us when we got off the bus in their neighborhood. We took the bus out of bustling San Miguel de Allende and made our way to a rural outpost half an hour away. You could easily see the church towers of the nearby city in one direction, but in the other direction it was dusty hillsides, dirt roads, and humble houses made of laminate or bricks. We got off the bus and looked around but did not see anyone. Alma got out her cell phone and called Rosa's mother, who told us just to walk to their house. "Just go down the hill to the cornfield, and you will see our house. It's the only one with two windows made of *tabique* (red bricks)," she told Alma—just as Alma's cell phone credit ran out. With those clues to go on, we gamely turned in circles looking around until we decided on a path that appeared most likely to arrive at what we thought might be a cornfield in the distance. On our way, we saw a man come out of his home with a large and scary dog who nearly pulled itself off the leash as it tried to get at us. Bravely, Alma called out to him to ask if he knew where Rosa, "the girl who just had a baby," lived, but he shook his head and yelled, "I don't know who you are talking about." We thanked him and quickly moved on but noticed that he stayed outside with his dog, watching us walk away.

"Obviously he knows who Rosa is and where she lives," Alma said, under her breath. "What do you mean?" I asked. "This is not a big neighborhood.

I am sure he knows her—he just doesn't want to tell us. They don't trust us, coming around in our uniforms," she explained. We did make a strange crew, two midwifery students in their pressed uniforms and backpacks and clipboards, accompanied by me with my notebook. "Later he will surely tell her, 'people were looking for you,' but he wants to protect her now because he doesn't know why we are here."

We walked on and found a house with two windows that seemed to fit the description, but nobody answered the door. We kept walking and found more houses that seemed right—none of them were Rosa's home. Finally, we saw a house with two windows, made partly of red brick and partly of laminate sheeting. It was only half built, but it was surrounded by a barbed-wire fence, and three dogs patrolled it, barking loudly from a small yard as we approached. A little boy peeked out to see what the commotion was, and Alma asked him to fetch his mom. The grandmother appeared instead and told us to come in. She walked us through the kitchen and living areas, which were unfinished with dirt floors, and into a bedroom—the only fully finished room in the house. There was a double bed in one corner, a makeshift bed of blankets on the floor, and a dresser overflowing with clothing and painted whimsically with flowers. A large table sat in the middle of the room with some snacks, baby formula, and rubbing alcohol on top. On the floor, amid the blankets, was a jumble of kittens curled up around a dirty diaper. Scraps of toilet paper and bubble wrap littered the floor, and two toddlers ran around laughing and playing.

Rosa stood next to the bed, looking nonplussed at our arrival. Alma introduced us all, asked her consent for me to observe the visit, and told her that we were there to check her for the midwife, to make sure that she was recovering from the birth. Rosa nodded and wordlessly motioned toward the bed behind her. We all turned and noticed, for the first time, the bundle of blankets that was her newborn baby. Alma and Rosa sat down on either side of the baby, and Alma carefully unwrapped him and checked his vital signs, while Yolanda watched Alma carefully, learning from the more advanced student. Alma noted that the umbilical cord looked a little infected (it was wrapped in toilet paper), and told Rosa that she should be cleaning it with a little alcohol to make sure it healed properly. She showed Rosa how to do exercises with the baby, stretching and moving his limbs gently, then she opened the curtains to get some more light as she continued to examine him. With more light, she realized that his face was slightly yellow, and she told Rosa to make sure that if his body got more yellow, to take him to the clinic. Throughout the exam, Rosa did not say much, but nodded and looked on as her older children ran in and out, trying to make us laugh.

Alma completed her examination, wrapped the baby back up, and turned to Rosa, asking her, "How are *you* doing?" In a quiet voice, Rosa replied that she was doing fine. Alma probed more deeply, asking if Rosa was always as pale as she appeared to be that morning. "Well, it may be from the hemorrhage I had after the birth," Rosa said casually. "Hemorrhage?" Alma asked, looking up in surprise. She did not have that in her notes. "Yes, the day after the birth, I was having headaches after that, and I felt like I couldn't really feel my body. The midwife sent me to get some medicine, and now I feel fine," Rosa explained, gesturing to bottles of chlorophyll juice and vitamins on the side table. Alma looked concerned, and took Rosa's temperature to make sure that she did not have any infection. Then she asked her how she was feeling, emotionally. "Do you have any support here?" Rosa said she was fine, that her mother helped out and her cousin came sometimes with her children. On cue, two children ran into the room, spilling candies and then sprawling on the floor to eat them. A dog wandered in and tried to eat the candies, and the kids shooed it away. Alma took advantage of the interruption to gently remind Rosa that she should not let the animals get too close to the baby, and that she and the children should wash their hands before touching him, as well.

The baby began to cry, so Alma asked if she could observe Rosa breastfeeding to make sure it was going well. Rosa sat back on the bed and began to nurse the baby, and after watching for a few minutes, Alma said they were doing great. "I didn't have milk at first, so I started giving him formula," said Rosa, gesturing to the tin of formula on the table. "It's normal not to have much milk at first," Alma assured her, adding that "everything you have at first is perfect for the baby's tiny stomach." Finally, Alma asked if the woman wanted any more children, to which Rosa replied that she did not. She had already talked to the midwife about her contraceptive options and would return to CASA at some point to figure it out.

Alma finished up her notes on Rosa and the baby, and we packed up and said goodbye to the family. The children and dogs followed us out, barking and laughing and waving to us as we made our way back up the road, past the cornfield, and quickly past the home of the unfriendly neighbor with the scary dog. As we walked, we discussed Rosa's case. There seemed to be no men present in the home, and we talked about how many men in this area had left to find work elsewhere. They returned and sent money home when they could, Alma noted, in a pattern that could be seen in the stalled completion of the home and in the spacing of the children. I asked Alma if she was worried about Rosa's conditions—her pallor, her baby's umbilical cord and yellow hue, her malaise about getting follow-up care, her household—but Alma just sighed and said, "At least we found her and made contact; at least I was able to examine her and the baby." Alma thought that they would be ok, but she would pass along her notes to the staff midwife back at CASA to see what next steps should be taken. We had come today because Rosa had missed her follow-up visit, so Alma worried aloud that Rosa may not come back to be seen if things got worse for her or the baby.

"The people don't trust health-care workers," explained Alison Bastien, an anthropologist, retired midwife, and teacher at CASA's school, when I related the story of this home visit to her some days later. "They don't believe that follow-up care can be free, and they don't always want people coming into their space. That's why they often won't let the student in, even if they go all the way to their doors." Alison brought up two important details in her observation. First, she referenced a latent mistrust in the health-care system. Second, concerns about and confusion over the economics of health care made many people wary to seek it out. Both issues contribute to poor outcomes, and, I argue, both stem from a legacy of infrastructural violence that has created the conditions by which women are not always able to get the care they need. For the midwives and midwifery students out pounding the pavement, searching out patients like Rosa, the job was doubly difficult: they had to show women that the way care is provided could be different, while also proving that they were the right ones for the job.

Other CASA students discussed this dual responsibility and their individual struggles with it. One afternoon during a CASA class on gender (which was being taught by two third-year students who had some background training on the topic), the students were wrapping up a viewing of the (then-recent) film *Orgasmic Birth: The Best Kept Secret* (Pascali-Bonaro 2008). In the movie, notable US experts like Ina May Gaskin (whose birth commune in Tennessee largely spawned the home-birth movement) and anthropologist Robbie Davis-Floyd talk about natural birth and contrast it with hospital birth. Notably, the film profiles some women who claim that they experienced physical pleasure during their peaceful home births. After the film, the students discussed what it would take for their patients to achieve such birthing environments (one student noted, for example, that the midwife herself had to remain calm, as her adrenaline levels could interfere with the birthing environment). Students started packing up their notebooks to leave, but then Luna, a second-year student, raised her hand and started to speak: "I do not see how this film is relevant here in Mexico," she said, causing everyone else to pause and listen. She explained, "Women here don't want to give birth in their houses. I've been to their houses; they are dirty and small, not fit for a home birth." All at once, other students began to push back, arguing that this was not a fair depiction. "What are you saying?" asked one student. "That poor women cannot have a home birth? The idea is to have the baby born in the atmosphere that it will be living in, and its home is clearly the best place for that." Luna considered this, then responded, "Yes, but culturally, people don't want to have their babies in a dirty home, with a donkey on one side and a pig on the other, when they could go to a clean hospital. So is it my job to convince them to have a home birth in these conditions?" Again, the other students clamored to respond, offended by Luna's depiction of their patients' homes. "You have it wrong," said one third-year student. "Your job is not to convince anyone to have a home birth. Your job is to convince *yourself* that a home birth is possible and often a good option but also to advocate for women to make their own decisions about where *they* want to give birth. Anyway, even if a woman's home does seem dirty or small, at every home birth I have attended, the woman has always made a nice clean space for her own birth. We have to trust women." Another third-year student nodded along and added to her classmate's argument:

> The women have to decide where they are going to give birth and how they will do it. Our job as midwives is to look for the tools and tell women what we have learned, from videos like the one we just watched. For example, I am stationed in the emergency room at the general hospital now for my clinical rotation, and the other day a woman came in at thirty-nine weeks, saying she was ready for her baby to be born. I told her that she still had time to go, that she could go home if she wanted, but she said no, that she was ready to have her baby. Then the doctor came and told her the same thing, but she did not want to go, so the doctor let her stay. To help the women we cannot just meet them in moments like that. We have to work with them for months leading up to that moment, to really understand their customs, backgrounds, past experiences, home life, culture, and desires. I want to know everything about a woman. It is not about convincing her to do anything; it is about listening and respecting her and making sure she has all the information to make her own decision, which I need to support.

For this student, the midwifery model of care revolved around the establishment of trust and mutual understanding with patients. This relationship was key to providing quality care that centered women's choices and prioritized their qualitative experiences, even amid a context in which resources were scarce. Their job, she was saying, was to advocate for women where they were—be it in small, crowded homes or in hospital wards. But as I heard throughout my research, their job was also about advocating for broader systemic changes that could improve conditions in homes and hospitals.

Humanizing the Infrastructure

During class one day at CASA's midwifery school, CASA founder Nadine held a special lecture for the students. She told them that, as activists for midwives nationwide, they all must be able to explain the history of Mexican midwives and justify their future profession. She told them a story to illustrate her point, a story I heard her tell over and over again to visiting politicians from across Mexico:

> The first state clinic to hire graduates from our school was in San Luis Potosi, deep in the Huasteca region of the state, where maternal mortality had been a big issue. After the CASA midwives began to work there, maternal mortality rates did not just fall—they fell to zero. The thing is, once women heard that the midwives were working at the clinic, they began to actually go there for their births instead of staying away. By bringing the women in to the clinic meant that they could get the care they need, from caring professionals: the professional midwives.

The midwives I worked with from across Mexico leveraged such success stories to argue that the very health-care system that had long pushed them out of its hospitals should welcome them back as authorities in the field of reproduction. Their selling points were multiple: midwives could practice in the marginalized, rural areas where doctors often could not—or would not—go. While other medical professionals would staff rural clinics for their year of service and then settle at more lucrative and comfortable urban positions, midwifery students were being recruited specifically from rural regions and prepared to return to their communities to provide care. Midwives also argued that they were more culturally sensitive to the needs of diverse women and could gain their trust enough to get them the services they need. In spreading these messages, they were making the case that midwives could mediate the conditions that prevented women from getting good care while also reconditioning women to trust health-care providers and expect better care.

Professionalized midwifery education in Mexico is in its early stages, and as such it is able to incorporate the most up to date of international norms for best practices and evidence-based approaches in its new curricula. In this way, midwives distinguish themselves from those in the health-care system who are increasingly called out for failing to meet such standards. In all these ways, midwives are attempting to recast midwifery as a strategy for national development rather than a symbol of Mexico's underdeveloped past.

It isn't just the midwives themselves who are advocating for midwifery to become part of the formal health-care system. Some prominent politicians are taking notice of the promise of midwifery for achieving maternal mortality reduction. During a midwifery conference in 2010, a representative from the Mexican National Institute of Public Health told the midwives that "90 percent of women who are going to hospitals are not getting the best care possible. The way for them to get better care, and to also reduce maternal mortality, is to include alternative providers like midwives." This link between including midwives in the system and improving care was attributed to the supposed innate ability of midwives to connect culturally to the needs of their patients, to the specific kinds of training midwives received, and to the failings of medical education in obstetrics.

Juan Luis Mosqueda Gómez, then secretary of health for the state of Guanajuato, reiterated that idea during a speech he gave to CASA midwifery students. Midwives, he said, offer something to improve the health-care system that "goes beyond the technical knowledge, the knowledge of skills they can do—it is emotional accompaniment in pregnancy and birth and also all the work of sensitization and education about the next pregnancy, family planning, lactation; all of this together is really what favors the reduction of maternal and infant mortality."

For the midwives I have worked with, contemporary Mexican midwifery represents a turning point. Their own national government has come to see its spotty attempts at occasional traditional-midwifery training workshops as largely futile and ultimately ineffective in improving the health of women who do not have access to biomedical reproductive health care. The international sphere began in the last two decades to gather evidence in the effort of convincing national governments that professional midwifery training is the way to go (UNFPA 2006)—a project which requires not only an investment in educational development and implementation but also a shift in political and professional attitudes toward midwives. As Mexico thus begins to shift its position from one that explicitly marginalizes midwives to one that supports the certification of midwives and employs them in its state clinics, Mexican midwives are taking on new roles. They are coming face to face with hospital obstetrics, participating in policy decisions regarding standards for midwifery training, and working alongside biomedical personnel charged with turning the country's maternal mortality numbers around.

Like newly minted doctors and other health-care providers in Mexico, CASA's midwifery graduates are also sent to complete a year of service in these government health centers (a process that many students described to me as quite scary yet fulfilling). However, CASA founder Nadine argued that this year of service was very different for the midwives and the doctors. The midwives, she said, often ended up using the time to train the nurses and doctors there in the humanized birth techniques they had practiced throughout their time at CASA, while the doctors spent the year getting hands-on experience for the first time. When I spoke with CASA graduates who were returning from their year of service, some described a similar experience: upon beginning their service, they were mistrusted or misunderstood—but by the end of their service, they were teaching everyone else the things they had learned at CASA. They were doing the work of simultaneously changing the conditions for women in health-care centers nationwide and changing the perceptions around midwifery as a profession.

One afternoon while waiting for patients in her consult room, Julieta, a practicing professional midwife at CASA and an alumna of its program, told me in detail about the year of social service she had to do in order to get her cédula professional.[4] For Julieta's post, she was sent a day's drive north of San Miguel de Allende to a state-run health clinic that had just finished hosting a previous CASA graduate and was therefore not unfamiliar with the new professional midwives. "I had never left my family before," recalled Julieta, "and when my brother took me up there I was very scared and very sad." The plan had been to get there while the other CASA graduate was still there so that she could show her the ropes; they arrived late, however, and missed each other by hours. Julieta told her brother that he had best just leave her there and not stay with her, "otherwise I said that I might just try to go home with him if I lost my resolve!" She waited alone for hours until the director could talk with her. "He told me I had some big shoes to fill, that the last CASA student had been amazing, and so they expected no less of me. In fact, he told me that they expected more!" While the director's words showed a support for midwifery that comforted Julieta, it also left her feeling the pressure of her new position.

Julieta was put to work immediately when a woman came in already in active labor. Julieta had to learn the system of that clinic quickly, with nurses and medical interns shouting at her and throwing scrubs and booties at her (items she would not have worn in the CASA clinic). She awkwardly helped the woman onto the bed—a complicated contraption with cold metal stirrups, she said, that she had never used before—and stood by while the others put up a sterile field, another element she had not had much experience with for vaginal births. She delivered the baby quickly and was happy that nothing went wrong. Yet the stress of the change of pace and the pressure to learn new ways of practicing, combined with homesickness, left Julieta feeling overwhelmed and lost for weeks.

With time and work, though, things began to improve. "There was so much work to do, sometimes ten births in one day!" Julieta exclaimed. At this memory, we both looked bleakly around the quiet consult room where we sat talking in CASA's clinic. Unlike the busy health center where she had done her year of service, CASA was a private clinic and had been steadily losing patients to the free state hospital up the road during the time I was conducting research. Julieta missed the busy pace she had gotten used to during that year. "I basically lived in that clinic," she said. "I would try to leave sometimes, but if a woman came in, in labor, I would come right back. I never wanted to leave them!" As they got to know her, the nurses and doctors came to respect Julieta, and she them. The nurses would always make sure that she was brought food as she worked through the day and night. A devout Catholic, Julieta recalled feeling as if all of the blessings patients gave her made her incredibly fortunate. "Everyone blessed me!" she said, grinning.

Julieta asserted that such blessings were what allowed her to get through some difficult deliveries during that year. In one case, a woman arrived already pushing. Julieta had never met with her during her pregnancy and knew nothing about her. "Her belly was gigantic," remembers Julieta. "But then when the baby finally came out, it was so small, with a strangely flattened face. I panicked and called the doctor, who said it was fine—only a little squashed from the delivery." However, as Julieta prepared to deliver the placenta, she was surprised to see another baby come shooting out. "Everyone began shouting," she remembered. "The woman knew all along she was carrying twins but didn't want to tell us so that she would not get sent in for a cesarean! That second baby had been pushing on his little brother, which is why his face looked all squished." Vaginally delivering twins was not something Julieta had been trained to do (such cases were normally referred to the physician), yet she had done it.

"That was not the only complicated birth I ended up attending," she told me. "Once I had a woman come in, already fully dilated and ready to push. When I checked her, I realized that what I was feeling was too soft—it was the baby's bottom, not its head!" Again, delivery of breech babies was not something that the professional midwives were trained to do—like twin births, this was a case to be referred to first-level hospitals. But again, in this case the woman was already pushing, and Julieta was put in charge. "I remembered that you cannot touch the baby with your skin, or pull on it as it comes out," Julieta said, "so that it doesn't try to start breathing, or arch its neck and get stuck in the pelvis." Terrified, she guided the baby out gently and slowly with a warm cloth, and mother and baby were both fine.

The nurses and medical interns grew to respect Julieta and her work as a midwife, *because* of her ability to use techniques that they had not learned through their biomedical training. Not completely aware of the impression that she could make within that biomedical setting, Julieta unabashedly employed techniques she had learned at CASA, such as using the *rebozo* (shawl) to help position babies or prescribing homeopathic medicines to her patients. She came to find out that some of the doctors had used homeopathic medicines with their patients before but always in secret—they did not want to be seen using such alternative remedies. "But once they realized how much people liked the homeopathic remedies I was using, even the other doctors started asking me for the ones I had to use on their patients, too!"

Julieta's experiences in her year of service gave her the confidence to employ the traditional and alternative midwifery techniques that she was more comfortable using, alongside or instead of the biomedical techniques that had structured her formal education at CASA. She was initially surprised by the medical staff's acceptance of her use of homeopathy and uterine massage, but she came to see that many of the biomedical practitioners themselves felt comfortable using alternative therapies due to their own previous exposure to them. As Byron Good and Mary-Jo Del Vecchio Good (1993, 83) point out, too often anthropological studies of medical practices tend to view them as homogenous entities. Within biomedicine, for example, they point out that practitioners do not all think or practice exactly the same, and details such as subspecialties or geographic locations dramatically alter the face of biomedicine. Julieta's experiences reveal how sometimes surprising approaches to care can emerge and make sense in settings where infrastructures and trust in medicine have been eroded.

Conclusion

The midwives I talked to often sounded defeated when they talked about the changes they wanted to make in the Mexican health-care system. There were so few of them, and it was such a large country, and the road was quite uphill. I understood their frustration and felt their concern—how could such a small group of women help so many in need while simultaneously changing the national perception of midwifery? Yet between their moments of frustration, the midwives told stories of triumph, and over time their stories and their statistics began to add up. They began to paint a picture of midwifery as a stopgap to the failings of infrastructure. They began to illustrate how they could bridge the needs of the population with the needs of the state: that is, to help women survive and thrive while helping reduce maternal mortality. And they did not require new roads to get there—just a few years of systematic training, a government certification, and a chance to work while making a decent living. They were trying to build themselves into the health-care system in a sustainable way.

And yet, even as the midwives tried to find ways to work with the system, they simultaneously pushed back against it. The midwives' critique of the current health-care system centered on a paradox: safe motherhood is supposed to be about getting women to hospitals, yet many women become unsafe if and when they get there. Women are conditioned to expect poor conditions. Stories like Irma's illustrate the stakes involved if hospitals are indeed unsafe spaces for birth. The personnel's mistreatment of Irma, and her subsequent unassisted birth on the patio, point to a system in need of change. The midwives I worked with argued that we must look beyond the assumed superiority of biomedical practitioners and institutions and appreciate the possibilities offered by an investment in midwifery for improving women's health outcomes. Indeed, their very training instilled in them from the start a need to embrace this dual role: to become part of the system while pushing for systemic change.

In the next chapter, I look more closely at another way that Mexican midwives pushed back against the health-care system, through an examination of their critiques of what they called "obstetric violence." Like the crumbling roads and crumbling trust in institutions described above, obstetric violence must be understood within a broader context of systemic failures that put women at risk. That is, the violence that the midwives described had become part of the maternal conditions in Mexico, which in turn had become part of the infrastructure. As midwives tried to critically address obstetric violence, they revealed the underlying failures that allowed it to become routinized across the country.

CHAPTER 4

Obstetrics in a Time of Violence

Midwives occupy a unique middle space between the Mexican state and its health-care facilities and the women and communities they serve. Like many of their patients, midwives have long been marginalized in the eyes of the state (Dixon, El Kotni, and Miranda 2019). Even as they slowly regain some authority in the realm of birth, they remain outsiders, and their gaze remains critical: they see things differently because they themselves are different in the eyes of the system. One of the things that their positionality allows them to notice is how violent the system can be. In previous chapters, I have talked about how infrastructural violence creates the built conditions for inequality and suffering (through bad roads, understaffed clinics, or a lack of radio repeater towers, for example) and how global health initiatives meant to improve health outcomes can do violence when they focus on numerical targets instead of holistic, quality care.

Here, I show how midwives have built a critique against health care in Mexico by arguing that broken infrastructure, entrenched gender inequality, and the unnecessary or dangerous medicalization of childbirth has led to the poor health outcomes that the country is struggling with. However, while such critiques echo the sentiments of feminist scholarship denouncing the medicalization of women's bodies, the framework the midwives use differentiates them: the term *violencia obstétrica* (obstetric violence) is being used by many Mexican midwives to describe hospital-based obstetric practices. By reframing obstetric practices as violent—as opposed to simply medicalized—these midwives seek to situate their concerns about women's health care in Mexico within regional discussions about violence, gender, and inequality.

While obstetric violence is an evocative concept, its insertion into social and legal systems has proven difficult, a symptom of the nascent and multifaceted nature of both the obstetric violence and midwifery movements in Mexico. While the term itself is not new, and the idea of creating legislation to criminalize acts of obstetric violence has been borrowed, Mexican midwives use the term in part to refer to structural modes of violence that are not always explicitly physical or easily codified and regulated. Their goal becomes twofold: to define and regulate specific obstetric practices in terms of overt violence and violation (infringements of rights) and to bring attention to deeper patterns of inequality and violence that play out in hospital delivery rooms. These goals distinguish the movement from earlier and ongoing attempts to "humanize" birth that address medicalization as a set of protocols to be changed. However, by attempting to address obstetric violence both as a set of physically violent practices and as a deeper structural concern, the midwives have come up against a question that anthropologists have also been debating in recent years: how can structural inequality on a broader scale be linked to tangible instances of physical violence? I argue that as midwives reflect on the violence they observe within hospitals and grapple with this question, what they try to articulate is that structural violence *is* physical violence; a common phrase linked to the movement argues that *violencia obstétrica* es *violencia de genero* (obstetric violence *is* gendered violence).

In this chapter I look closely at the emergence of the movement against obstetric violence as a socio-political concept and think about what it means alongside midwives' other critiques of the health-care system and their own career aspirations. Through their everyday experiences working with Mexican public hospitals and gaining clinical skills, midwives come to think about medicalization and violence in interesting ways. How do Mexican midwives define incidences of violence in obstetric settings, and what work does this definition do for women's health and for midwifery as a profession that stands in contrast to biomedical obstetrics? How and to what end do they come to push back against the system they simultaneously work within? My research shows that as midwives come together and do the work of defining and theorizing obstetric violence, they seek to bring attention to the topic of medicalized birth in a way that reflects particular constellations of gender, power, history, and biomedicine in Mexico today. This approach does work that the humanized birth movement has not been able to do, by tapping into timely concerns about violence in other realms of Mexican society and by shifting the responsibility for medical choices in birth away from patients and onto providers and health-care systems.

The topic of obstetric violence has emerged alongside three broader conversations among academic and activist circles: feminist critiques of the medicalization of women's health, typologies of violence, and violence in Latin America. Feminist anthropologists have traced the effects of medicalization and hypermedicalization—which refers to the overuse or misuse of biomedical intervention—on women's bodies and reproductive health. While I argue here that the obstetric violence movement attempts to move beyond these critiques of medicalization, its understandings of power and authority in biomedicine are anchored in such feminist critiques. For decades, scholars have been discussing distinctions between physical, symbolic, and structural violence (Galtung 1969, 1990; Farmer 1996), yet debates continue over how these distinctions map onto lived experiences (Goldstein 2007; Nichter and Medeiros 2015). I show how this academic debate plays out in a parallel fashion within the midwifery community in Mexico, as midwives struggle to make the term "obstetric violence" fit as a descriptor for both overt physical violence and deeper structural violence against women. Finally, I situate obstetric violence within conceptions of violence in Latin America and Mexico in particular. Bringing attention to obstetric violence becomes a way for the midwives to talk about normalized violence related to gender, class, and race in Mexico more generally; as Philippe Bourgois argues, such "intimate violence" is increasingly replacing the more overt political violence across Latin America, and in its path it "has legitimated social inequality and demobilized popular demands for the redistribution of resources" (2010, 18). However, within Mexico the recent explicit demonstrations of violence connected to drug cartel tensions have made violence an everyday word. Might the obstetric violence movement draw on these tensions in its attempt to bring attention to gendered violence that plays out in hospitals nationwide?

Evidence within Bodies

The manifestations of obstetric violence are sometimes subtle and hard to see, accounting in part for the difficulty faced by the midwives trying to bring attention to them. I was observing with students at CASA's professional midwifery school and clinic in San Miguel de Allende, Guanajuato, one morning when a patient came in bearing the evidence of such hidden violence within her body. It was a slow day in the clinic, and two students were assisting Ana, the staff midwife, during a routine women's health exam.

The patient—a young woman from a nearby *rancho* (rural community)—had come in alone. She spoke quietly, explaining that she was worried something was wrong with her uterus. Cancer, maybe—she didn't know. When Ana asked why she thought that, the patient explained that she had been trying to get pregnant with a second child for a year now, but to no avail.

"I was taking birth control pills since my last birth," she explained, "but I stopped them a year ago, and I still haven't gotten pregnant. Something must be wrong." Ana assured her that this was normal but told her that she and her students would examine her to ensure that she was healthy. While the patient undressed in the bathroom, the midwife turned to her students to explain that pregnancy can sometimes take many months and that this is not necessarily cause for alarm. The patient emerged in a blue hospital gown and lay down on the exam table. With Ana guiding her, one of the students explained carefully as she prepared to conduct a pap smear and pelvic exam. She was part of the way through when she looked up at Ana and exclaimed that the woman had an intrauterine device (IUD), a long-term form of birth control that is inserted into the uterus. Ana finished the exam, shaking her head in frustration. It turned out that the doctor at the general hospital had inserted the IUD immediately after her first baby was born, without her consent.[1] This meant that she had been taking birth control pills for years unnecessarily and explained why she failed to get pregnant even a year after she stopped taking them. The patient was surprised at the news but also happy to have an explanation for her fertility concerns. She scheduled an appointment to get the IUD removed during her next period. Once she left, the midwife and her students expressed their outrage.

"The problem is not only the lack of consent when doctors put IUDs in immediately postpartum," Ana told her students. "It is also that they shouldn't even put them in that soon—the uterus is not ready for that yet![2] But when women have their babies at the hospital, the doctor almost always puts one in, whether she wants it or not. Sometimes they tell women, 'you can always get it out later, let me just put it in now.'" The students concurred; while completing their professional midwifery degree at CASA, they conducted clinical rotations at the local public hospital. While there, they witnessed the coercive use of IUDs on a daily basis and were increasingly frustrated by their inability to stop the practice. "On top of that," exclaimed one student, "the hospitals make it nearly impossible for the women to get the IUDs removed later—they don't want these women having any more babies!" The others nodded their heads, saying that they saw many patients here at CASA who wanted their IUD removed because their doctor at the hospital would not take it out. "This is violence and violation!" exclaimed Ana. For Ana and her students, the violence committed against their patients happened on many registers; it was present in the lack of consent, in the coercive use of the IUD, in the refusal to help women, and in the general attitude toward women's bodies and their fertility. Here, violence was also seen in their patient's unwitting consumption of birth control pills on top of the protection of the IUD that she was not aware she carried in her uterus. Ana and her students used the term "obstetric violence" to describe what they saw happening at the hospital. Yet this term does more than catalogue individual inhumane practices: it seeks to reframe them as the indicators of pervasive, underlying gendered violence.

Medicalization, Hypermedicalization, and Humanization

When midwives like Ana and her students talk about practices like the coercive use of IUDs as cases of obstetric violence, they reference two distinct but related sets of conditions. First, they critique the routine technologies and infrastructures that have developed within biomedical settings by calling out their unnecessary or improper usage. Second, they critique the less easily codified, and more insidious, incidences of violence that occur between providers and patients that they see as indicative of trends in social violence toward women. Indeed, scholarship on obstetric violence has increasingly recognized what the midwives were trying to describe— that obstetric violence is gender violence, that it is violence against women because they are women (Cohen Shabot 2016). In this section, I differentiate between critiques of medicalization and hypermedicalization in order to contextualize obstetric violence within scholarly and activist movements related to obstetric care.

The arguments made about the mechanisms behind and effects of the medicalization of childbirth echo a large body of feminist scholarship from recent decades (Mitford 1992; Arms 1975; Martin 1987; Rich 1976; Katz Rothman 1991). Building on Foucault's (1973) notion of the "clinical gaze," such scholars have highlighted specific ways that female bodies come under scrutiny as objects of study and how reproductive processes from menstruation to menopause (and everything in between) have consequently been pathologized. Once reproductive processes are defined solely in terms of medical problems, scholars argue, they must be managed and treated with biomedical interventions (Riessman 1983). As technological intervention into all reproductive processes proliferates, "normal" reproduction becomes classified increasingly as a dangerous throwback, which could detract from women's ability to achieve perfection as feminine bodies and mothers. In fact, what counts as "normal" is itself being redefined; as Davis-Floyd and Dumit (1998, 9) point out, for example, technology in childbirth has become so naturalized that now a hospital birth with any number of biomedical interventions is being called "natural," in opposition only to cesarean births. As conceptions of what counts as normal are shifted by technological interventions in childbirth, the potential for new kinds of bodies is created.

While medicalization thus relates to the gradual redefinition of bodily processes as medical domains, scholarship focusing on hypermedicalization explicitly emphasizes the overuse or misuse of medicine and technology in health care. Studies pointing toward the negative health impacts of hypermedicalized childbirth, such as its correlation with high cesarean section rates (Simonds, Rothman, and Norman 2006) and its inability to lower maternal mortality rates in developing countries, have inspired calls for investigations into the specific manifestations of medicalization in diverse childbirth settings (Boddy 1998). That is, how practitioners approach birth and what women experience must both be understood within the political and social contexts of specific times and places (Ginsburg and Rapp 1995). In particular, scholars have called for more work on the impacts of the uneven exportation of medicalized childbirth in developing countries as a reflection of unequal distributions of power related to gender, race, class, and nationality. By looking at moments of hegemonic imposition of medicalized childbirth techniques within specific contexts of development, we may be able to see beyond manifestations of structural violence to understand the grounded motivations and mechanisms by which childbirth becomes a contested process.

Anthropologists have argued that it is equally important to address moments of resistance to hypermedicalized birth in diverse settings and to consider who is resisting and how they delineate their concerns. Scholars have looked at midwifery as a site for the promotion of a model of care that stands in opposition to the hypermedicalization of birth (Davis-Floyd 2001b; Simonds, Rothman, and Norman 2006). The humanized birth movement, which was popularized for Latin America during the First International Humanization of Birth Conference in Brazil in 2000 (Page 2001), has sought to unite patients, midwives, doctors, and activists alike to call for

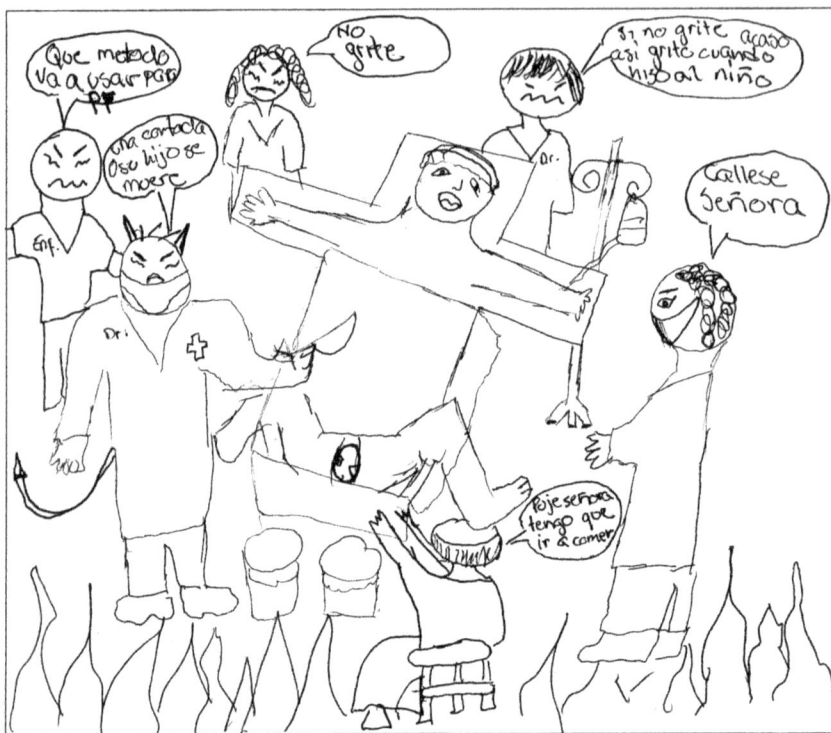

FIGURE 5: A midwifery student's drawing of her perception of birth in a Mexican public hospital.

an analysis of the overuse of unnecessary interventions and technologies in birth. In Mexico, midwives have taken up the call to "humanize" birth, a project they say is founded on the notion that birth is a normal event in which women should be in charge, and medical interventions should be used only when necessary (Alonso and Gerard 2009). Despite their promotion of the benefits of humanized childbirth, however, increasing pressure by free state health programs has pushed more women than ever into the hypermedicalized system and the very circumstances that midwives are trying to change.

Midwifery students drew clear connections between the unnecessary use of medical interventions and the mistreatment of women in hospital obstetrics. In fact, after hearing so many students describe to me their discomfort or outright anger with what they saw as obstetric violence disguised as medical care, I asked them to draw for me what this looked like to them. I asked students at CASA as well as at the Mujeres Aliadas professional

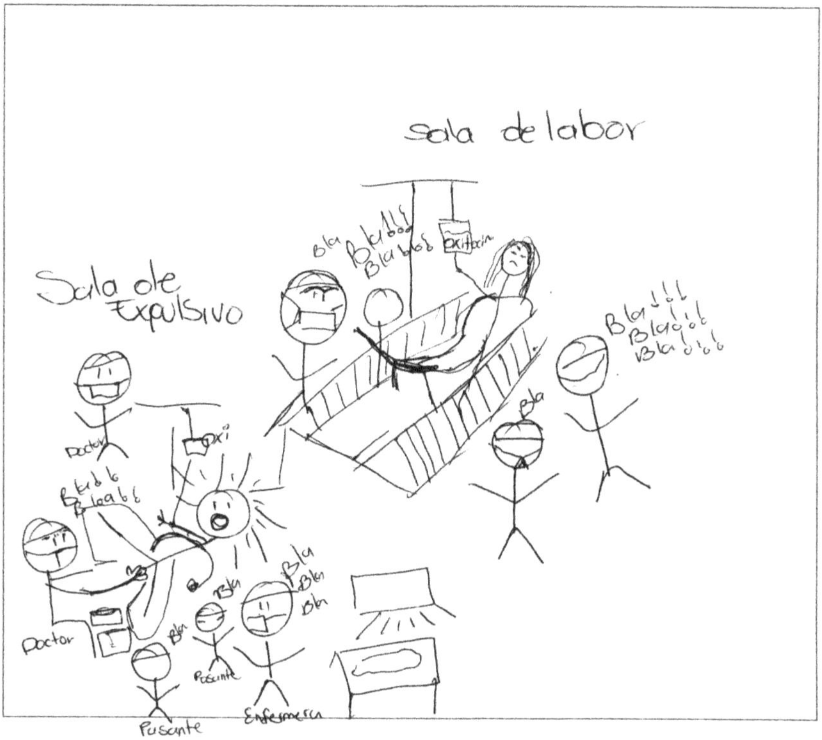

FIGURE 6: A midwifery student's drawing of two female patients and assorted medical professionals in a public hospital labor room and delivery room.

midwifery school in Pátzcuaro, Michoacán, to draw pictures of birth from their perspective, first in the hospital obstetrics wards where they worked or conducted clinical rotations, then in their idealized, midwifery-led settings (see Dixon 2020 for a more thorough discussion of this exercise as a method in ethnographic fieldwork).[3] The drawings became touch points for further analysis and conversation and allowed students to more clearly visualize the ways that hypermedicalization could be interpreted as obstetric violence.

Figures 5, 6, and 7 are representative of the ways that students drew patient-provider interactions in the hospital setting. In Figure 5, a woman labors seemingly among the fires of hell, while a doctor—drawn to look like a devil—warns her that "one little cut or your baby dies." The doctor receiving the baby says, "Push, lady—I have to go eat." The other staff compel her to shut up; one asks the question that so many students reported hearing repeated in hospital wards: "Is this how you yelled when you made the baby?" This kind of humiliating, often sexually tinged scolding has been well documented across Mexico and beyond (see, for example: El Kotni 2018; Bohren et al. 2019; Brink 2019; Smith-Oka 2015). Even the nurse asking about the patient's family-planning desires appears aggressive: "What method are you going to use for family planning?" she asks, with her face drawn in an angry scowl (again, an attitude and pervasive topic of questioning in Mexican obstetrics wards; see El Kotni 2018). Figure 6, similarly, shows women being yelled at ("bla bla bla!!!" read the captions, indicating the meaninglessness of the things they are yelling at women) as they grimace in pain in the labor and delivery areas of the hospital. In these artistic depictions, we can see how the problem here is not a lack of medical care or attention; this patient is fully attended to, at least physically. All the tools of biomedical childbirth are represented—the bed, the IV, the scalpel, the fully staffed delivery room. The problem is the violence and aggression seemingly directed toward her, which we see reflected back to us in the patient's scared, vulnerable body language.

Many of the students' drawings included such elements with a similar message—that the tools of medicine can become the tools of torture when employed in inhumane and unnecessary ways. Indeed, in Figure 7, when asked to draw birth in the public hospital, the student focused solely on the interventions and medications involved: birth is represented here by a container of the drug Pitocin (labeled here as *oxitocina*), a syringe, an IV bag, and drawers of medications. The humanity that enters into the image is truncated. One speech bubble says, "Push, lady, push . . ." In the upper right corner, we see a hand going toward a vagina, with "*tacto*!!" (the term used to describe the manual checking of cervical dilation, something that students reported as being done too frequently and roughly on laboring women).[4] The woman appears only from the point of view of the receiving practitioner—we see her legs open, her perineum cut and bleeding, and that she is exclaiming, "Aah!"

Not all of the midwives and midwifery students I worked with had such hospital-based, clinical exposure; for some, their concerns about obstetric violence stemmed from their own personal negative experiences or from the stories they heard from their patients and communities. But the increasing presence of midwives and their students in state health-care facilities meant that they were seeing such violence first hand, over and over again. It wore on them, it wore them down, and it made them feel incredibly helpless and angry. But it also lent energy to their campaign to name the violence they

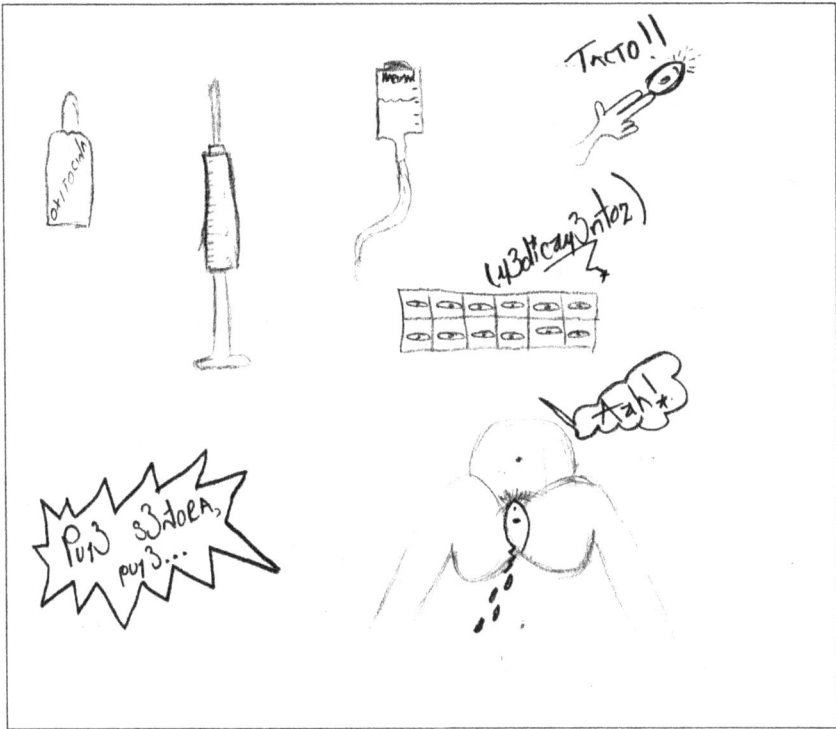

FIGURE 7: A midwifery student's drawing of the tools of birth in a public hospital setting.

saw and to advocate for systemic changes that might lead to real change in the way women were treated. Once again, midwives acted from their middle ground as representatives of health care charged with improving health outcomes and as advocates for women and for systemic change.

Naming and Framing Obstetric Violence

By 2019, the term "obstetric violence" had become much more recognized in Mexico and worldwide, as stories of abuses women faced during labor spread across social media and were taken up by news sources, and lawmakers began to incorporate the term into state and national legislation. The National Human Rights Commission (CNDH) in Mexico explicitly linked obstetric violence to both gender violence and structural violence and has pushed for the past few years for increased legislation to address it—including the inclusion of midwives in the health-care system. During my fieldwork, I witnessed the first rumblings about the term and saw from the start how its insertion into legislation and practice proved tricky. I also saw how midwives took up the term early on, as it resonated with the specific kinds of institutional, gender-based violence they witnessed in public hospitals and heard about from their patients.

In 2011, Nueve Lunas traditional midwifery school in the Mexican state of Oaxaca sent out a mass email as part of a campaign to change Oaxacan law to include obstetric violence within other forms of violence against women that the state was responsible for policing. The document—which was sent to policymakers, activists, midwives, and academics nationwide— was titled, "The need to generate a scientific and rational debate to categorize obstetric violence as gendered violence: Pronouncement of organizations from the civil society." It argued: "Obstetric violence is a reality that must be legislated! Never again should women have a life with violence!" Obstetric violence was situated squarely within conversations about both gendered violence against women and national concerns over maternal mortality. Obstetric violence, it said, is distinct from other kinds of violence that have become more publicly visible in recent years. "Obstetric violence has remained hidden and silenced," it read. Yet, "the lack of quality in the attention to pregnancy and birth has been shown to be one of the principal factors responsible for maternal mortality and morbidity, along with discrimination based on gender, ethnicity, race, and class." The document went on to blame the violation of sexual and reproductive rights, along with a lack of universal access to health services, for Mexico's continuing problems with maternal health outcomes.

The document linked concerns about obstetric violence to multiple international scientific sources, while also situating this newly conceptualized violence within Latin America's historical legacies of violence and social movements (Caldeira 2002; Eckstein 2001). Oaxacan midwives were not the first to propose legislative changes based on the term, however; the Mexican state of Veracruz had, three years before, promised women a "life free of violence"—including obstetric violence (Calzada Martinez 2009). One year before that, Venezuela had set the precedent in Latin America by rendering obstetric violence illegal (Pérez D'Gregorio 2010). According to Venezuelan law, obstetric violence was defined as: "the appropriation of the body and reproductive processes of women by health personnel, which is expressed as dehumanized treatment, an abuse of medication, and to convert the natural processes into pathological ones, bringing with it loss of autonomy and the ability to decide freely about their bodies and sexuality, negatively impacting the quality of life of women" (Pérez D'Gregorio 2010, 201). For both Veracruz and Venezuela, markers of obstetric violence included such infractions as forcing women to give birth lying down, denying women timely emergency obstetric care, and performing cesarean sections when not medically indicated. The Venezuelan law also set the punishment: practitioners convicted of such acts of violence would be charged a fee, and the practitioner and his or her institution must sign a copy of the given sentence, thus ensuring institutional accountability (Pérez D'Gregorio 2010).

The laws passed in Venezuela and Veracruz were and continue to be novel in their attempt to hold health practitioners legally accountable to international norms and recommendations about best practices in obstetrics. However, a year after the law was passed in Veracruz, no lawsuits had arisen —a fact blamed on the lack of general knowledge about the law and even about the concept of obstetric violence (Calzada Martinez 2009). Similarly, in Venezuela, a follow-up article published in 2011 of a study conducted in multiple national hospitals revealed that, while the term *violencia obstétrica* was widely known, and many practitioners reported seeing instances of violence inflicted on patients there, paths for recourse and reporting were unknown, so little could be done for the victims (Faneite, Feo, and Toro Merlo 2012). The mounting humanitarian crisis in Venezuela, which led to massive shortages of health-care services and supplies (from blood to medications to sterile instruments) has, in recent years, led to skyrocketing maternal mortality rates and rapidly deteriorating conditions for care (Moloney 2019), such that many women have been streaming across the border into Columbia to give birth (Schaefer Muñoz 2017).

When the Oaxacan midwives sent out their email urging Mexican women to fight for a law that was similar to what Venezuela had at least passed (even if it has since become buried among other health-related concerns), their grievances with obstetric care were strikingly similar, perhaps because they were both drawing on international norms and recommendations. In fact, Mexico had already taken up many of these recommendations as its own in the national Official Norms outlined to help reduce maternal mortality. What the midwives were asking for, then, was a way to turn national recommendations into legal accountability; officials did not respond positively, however.

"Our proposal was shut down by the government," explained Marta, one of the administrators at Nueve Lunas school, as she gave me a tour of their facilities. "It was all because the doctors were pressuring them." Marta's explanation was echoed by a national journalist covering the issue, who noted that doctors saw the potential law as an effort to criminalize routine medical practice; doctors had argued that the law should not intervene in doctor-patient relationships (Mino 2012). For Marta and the rest of Nueve Lunas, this argument made little sense. Doctors were making it sound as if the midwives were saying that "any doctor or nurse who participated in a cesarean could go to jail, which is a lie and a manipulation" (Mino 2012; my translation). Despite official rejection, Marta continued, the idea of obstetric violence had been publicized more widely; she hoped that more women might at least come to realize that they had the right to a birth free of violence.

Something that stands out in both Nueve Luna's proposed law and in the Venezuelan legal depiction of obstetric violence is their very banality;[5] that is, the offensive practices listed in them reflect trends in the hypermedicalization of childbirth worldwide. The overuse of cesarean sections and the dependence on the supine position for delivery (that is, making women deliver while on their backs rather than in vertical positions), for example, have been long critiqued within the framework of unnecessary medicalization of childbirth (see Mitford 1992; Arms 1975; Katz Rothman 1991), yet this current movement reframes these and other such routine practices as indications of violence—not just less-than-ideal practices carried out by unknowing but well-meaning providers. I suggest that this reframing is strategic in that it aims to shift such practices from being merely unnecessary to being dangerous, as well as a direct reflection of practitioner and institutional attitudes to the women they serve.

Getting women and practitioners to question practices that are seen as technologically and biomedically superior has been difficult for the midwives, even as they argue that such practices do not always lead to better outcomes. The exportation of biomedical, Western techniques for birthing practices has often caused more harm than its model would predict. In many cases, the developing world has enthusiastically implemented biomedical modes of birth, such as making women labor on their backs, injecting them with high amounts of the drug Pitocin, not allowing them food or drink, etc. Yet these elements of labor were derived in settings where epidurals were being used commonly; in developing countries, epidurals are very often too expensive, so women are going through more painful labors than if they had been allowed to labor in other ways.

Bringing attention to the misuse or overuse of technological and biomedical interventions in childbirth is an important part of the obstetric violence movement, then; however, data from conversations with midwives and midwifery students from across Mexico suggests that, in bringing attention to bad practices, many midwives are also trying to bring attention to deeper gendered violence that plays out in delivery rooms. It is because of their newfound authority in women's health in Mexico that many midwives are now able to work in state clinics or hospitals; it is this same authority that has given them a platform from which to critique what they see. Implicit in this critique is their argument that midwifery care offers a non-violent—humanized—alternative in care.

Unnecessary Interventions

Students at the CASA midwifery school were learning clinical skills during rotations in public hospitals where they came face to face with multiple manifestations of obstetric violence. There was a strong ethos of activism within CASA's educational model, and students were told from early on that they were being primed to address not only issues of maternal mortality (although, as discussed in Chapter 2, they were also taught to frame their intervention in terms of its ability to address maternal mortality) but also of poor treatment of women. Further, CASA's students belonged to larger midwifery networks, such as those behind national efforts to bring attention to obstetric violence. As they reflected on their encounters with violence in hospitals, they emphasized most clearly an institutionalized pressure on doctors to continue bad practices in obstetrics, and they articulated these practices in terms of their violation of women's bodies, privacy, rights, and health. CASA students pointed to the unnecessary but compulsory use of episiotomies and Pitocin on nearly every hospital patient as examples of such violation.[6]

However, the hospital practice that students most frequently discussed in terms of violence and violation was the *revisión manual de cavidad uterina* (manual revision of uterine cavity), which they referred to more often as simply a *revisión de cavidad*. In the *revisión de cavidad*, the doctor manually scrapes out the woman's uterus (after delivery of the baby and placenta) with a gloved hand in order to make sure that no pieces of the placenta remain that could cause infection.[7] The World Health Organization has long listed this practice under those which are "Clearly Harmful or Ineffective and Should Be Eliminated" (WHO 1997, 122), and despite its routine use in Mexico since the 1960s, studies have repeatedly shown its inability to reduce the postpartum hemorrhage and highlighted the iatrogenic risks that the procedure itself entails (Sachse-Aguilera and Calvo-Aguilar 2013). During interviews about their experiences in public hospitals, students and practicing midwives across Mexico described this routine medical procedure as one of the most offensive experiences women had to go through there, both because of the intense pain it can cause (it is done without anesthesia in most cases) and because of its lack of basis in evidence as a preventative measure.

At the public hospital where some of my midwifery student informants did their rotations, the *revisión de cavidad* was standard for nearly every birth. Despite seeing it performed so many times, the practice still deeply affected the student midwives, and they talked about it often to each other, to their teachers, and to me. It was during such conversations in the time between shifts that students and midwifery teachers collectively articulated the parameters of obstetric violence. "It is horrible to watch the doctor do the manual revision," shuddered one of the third-year students as she described the procedure to some of the younger students while they waited for their teacher to arrive. "You can hear the doctor's fingers, scraping away at the woman. Often, the woman screams louder in that moment than when she was in labor. They do this even if the placenta came out totally intact!" Another student empathized, saying that,

> One time, it made sense to do the revision, because the placenta did not come out. But that was because the doctor had pulled on the cord so hard it broke, and so then he *had* to go in manually to retrieve the placenta! But other times, the placenta is obviously complete, and they still do it. I remember once an obstetric intern was there and saw the placenta come out, intact, and asked me—the midwifery student!—if he should do a manual revision. I said, "Why would you? You don't need to," and so he decided he wasn't going to do it. But then the attending physician came along and made him do it anyway. It is a matter of protocol (*protocolo*)!

Here, the intern and the midwife are both in a similar position of learning practices through the dominant protocols within which they are stationed. The midwife, however, must balance what she learns in the hospital with what she learns back in CASA's midwifery classes, while the intern will continue to depend on the attending hospital physicians for guidance. While students often referred to such individual physicians who resisted established hospital protocols—and indeed admired many local doctors as teachers, friends, and colleagues—doctors as a category were seen as part of the larger institutional problem. Vania Smith-Oka's (2013, 596) work on the misuse of cervical examinations in a Mexican public hospital reminds us to "contextualize, though not excuse" physicians' actions as part of the increasing bureaucratization of childbirth. Indeed, through conversations with doctors at the same hospital where students watched the *revisión de cavidad*, I came to better understand the context within which they were acting: many doctors had been taught that the *revisión* was vitally important to prevent infection, and they seemed genuinely concerned about the idea of sending their patients home to far-off rural communities without what they saw as an assurance of their well-being (this overshadowed any knowledge about recommendations against not doing the *revisión* without solid indications). They recognized that the procedure was painful but felt that the brief moments it took were worth the pain. While they acknowledged that the procedure should ideally be done under anesthesia, they noted that in hospitals like theirs, where one anesthesiologist had to run between the operating room, the emergency room, and the cesarean room, there was little possibility of getting anesthesia for women during this minor procedure. For all these reasons, the doctors just did not seem to understand why midwives would take such issue with this practice. The midwives, despite their increasing presence working within hospitals, maintained their positions as outside observers and saw the *revisión* as primarily a willful act of violence against women.

Elizabeth, a third-year midwifery student, grew angry as she described to her classmates her worst experience at the general hospital: "I was observing a birth with a doctor, who told me that I had to do the manual uterine revision on the patient myself," she said. "Her placenta had not come out intact, but that was because he had pulled it out before it was ready! I whispered to the doctor 'no,' that I would not do the revision, but the doctor told me I had to, so I stuck my hand in, but only up to the wrist, and checked the vaginal canal. Because I hadn't done it right, the doctor had to do it too." At this point, Elizabeth stretched out her arm in front of her, pointing to a spot about two inches up her forearm from her wrist to illustrate how far the doctor's arm was inserted. "The doctor went on to manually scrape out the remaining pieces of placenta," she said, shaking her head. In Elizabeth's view, if the doctor had allowed the placenta to emerge on its own, the patient would not have needed the *revisión de cavidad* in the first place. Yet because the placenta had broken, the doctor's actions were validated and necessary—the pieces of the placenta had to be taken out.

As with most obstetric procedures being critiqued in the obstetric violence movement (such as cesarean sections, episiotomies, or the use of coercive contraceptive techniques), many CASA midwives expressed the view that the technique of manually scraping out the uterus in search of remnants of a torn placenta has its place; as in the above story, where the placenta was not intact, it can be life-saving to prevent infection caused by such remnants. Sara, a CASA-trained professional midwife who taught at the school, told a group of students one afternoon about how all that observation of manual revision eventually helped her midwifery practice. Her brother had called her up one day to ask her to come help one of her mother's (also a midwife) patients. The woman had delivered the baby two hours prior, and the placenta had yet to emerge. The cervix was already closing, so Sara decided on the spot that she would have to manually dilate it and bring out the placenta with her hand, which was what she did. However, she was careful to differentiate the manner in which she did the *revisión de cavidad* to the students. By that point, she said, the placenta had become calcified and hard, attaching itself firmly to a spot on the uterine wall. Slowly, with minute and gentle finger movements, she unattached it and delivered it. In doing this, she told me, she possibly saved the woman's life. In her recounting, Sara highlighted the importance of not only having the practical know-how and the knowledge of when to use it but also approaching women in a respectful and gentle manner—thus distinguishing her usage of the technique from that of the doctors. In practice, it is hard to know how gentle the procedure felt to the patient, who did not have anesthesia. What Sara seemed to be stressing to her students, however, was that midwifery births may not be free from pain, but midwives can help women through that pain by treating them with care.

Tensions in the Movement, Tensions in the Concept

There is a tension in the movement against obstetric violence. The tension revolves around the dual meaning of the violence being discussed; on the one hand, there is a tangible and acute violent act being described, while on the other hand there is a chronic and systemic violence being alluded to. The midwives involved in efforts to legally regulate obstetric violence struggle with this tension, as do the midwifery students struggling to articulate their reactions to the everyday acts of violence they witness with their patients in the general hospitals. Will the regulation of specific obstetric practices be able to address the deeper gendered violence behind them?

This tension reflects the complexities involved in trying to address violence on multiple registers—from overt physical violence, in which there is a clear actor perpetrating an act of violence on a victim, to structural violence, in which there is no clear perpetrator, to cultural violence, which is any violence justified through cultural elements (Galtung 1969, 1990). While in the 1990s, the field of medical anthropology took up the notion of structural violence as a way to approach poverty and inequality from multiple perspectives and to demand political change on a larger scale (see Scheper-Hughes 1992; Farmer 1996; Biehl 2005), in more recent years there has been a backlash to such work. Within anthropology, critiques of the structural violence approach have taken two forms: one body of scholars argues that a focus on structural violence decenters culture from the analysis in favor of a less specific framing based on political economy; other scholars argue that the political project of the structural violence approach is too entangled with moral assumptions (Goldstein 2007). Can obstetric violence refer both to physical violence and to structural violence without erasing culture as a variable or making moral assumptions?

The obstetric violence movement positions specific obstetric practices within a framework of historical and ongoing patterns of social inequality, especially related to gender, race, and class. Indeed, recent scholarship on mistreatment in women's clinical encounters around the world has pointed to the importance of paying attention to the ways that these patterns of inequality intersect (Jewkes and Penn-Kekana 2015; Sadler et al. 2016; Davis 2019). How women are treated in labor and birth, the midwives argue, mirrors how they are treated in society in general. For many midwives, this means that women are set up from the beginning to be treated poorly in public hospitals—because of their status as lower class and/or Indigenous. As CASA founder Nadine put it, "It's not just that the system lets women die—it's that the system is built in ways that make women more likely to die. They set it up for you to die . . . then the government comes in to save you with interventions you wouldn't have needed had they just left you alone to start with." From her perspective, the failures in hospital care are allowed to perpetuate, then, because they are followed by what she sees as obstetric heroics. What if, asks the obstetric violence movement, these failures were addressed, and women could get better quality care from the start?

Many of the midwives in my study were aware of the historical legacies that underlie the inequalities they witnessed in hospital settings. During a midwifery class taught by two of the students, the topic turned to gender, race, class, and inequality in Mexico. One of the teachers, Alicia, told the students to read Octavio Paz's (1994) *The Labyrinth of Solitude* as a text which "explains why we Mexicans are *hijos de la chingada* (children of the fucked one): because we are all still the result of the Spanish fucking the Indigenous." Alicia, like Paz, argued that the legacy of the Spanish conquest of Mexico created inequalities that continue to shape social and political life in Mexico today. In doing this, she roots current inequalities in a certain ongoing inevitability, yet she also marks the significance of the work they are trying to do as midwives. The midwives' use of violence in their critique references this longer history of violation and abuse, while perhaps gaining a certain purchase in this moment because of more current invocations of violence in Mexican society.

To address obstetric violence on a national level means addressing the structural violence which perpetuates systems of inequality and abuse and which culminates in specific obstetric practices in public hospitals. While some midwives may be able to advocate for changes to the national norms and protocols, getting doctors to deploy these changes in their existing practices —and getting women to demand them—present a much bigger challenge. For both the doctors and their patients, recognizing current actions as forms of violence in need of redress would necessitate a reevaluation of the power dynamic between doctors and patients, which is connected to issues of class, race, gender, and poverty. Recent work in anthropology and health has begun to examine more closely the nuances of class, gender, race, and ethnicity within acts of violence and how such acts get inscribed on bodies. Such inscriptions are not necessarily dramatic and obvious—more often they occur in the mundane violence of the everyday (such as in the delivery room of a crowded public hospital) (Rylko-Bauer, Whiteford, and Farmer 2009). They are also not always so easily linked to individual actors, such as doctors or nurses; indeed, scholarship on medical racism in particular has shown how insidious acts of violence based on underlying inequalities may be, especially in reproductive health care, when "the medical complex, in each of its parts, cumulatively dismisses, misdiagnoses, and undermines women's feelings and intuitions about their reproducing bodies" (Davis 2019, xv).

In naming their movement as one that fights against obstetric violence, the midwives align themselves with a broader movement seen in anthropology that seeks to "recognize violence in the places where it is no longer recognized for what it is," which is often "in social processes that the dominant discourse never articulates in terms of violence" (Fassin 2009, 117). Yet the midwives, in this fight, are attempting not only to address issues of quality in maternal health care but rather to link quality of care issues to social concerns. In this goal, they put into action a strategy which has gained momentum within anthropology as well: through a critical examination of health, scholars hope to find new ways to confront global concerns related to inequality and violence (Rylko-Bauer, Whiteford, and Farmer 2009; Bourgois et al. 2017).

Violent Times

Even as midwives were crafting legislation and petitions against obstetric violence, they could not avoid discussions of other manifestations of violence in their surroundings. During the time this research was conducted, news related to drug cartels and the violence surrounding them was ever present and was affecting many who were unconnected to the cartels. While I was visiting Nueve Lunas, a traditional midwife named Carmelita had come to lecture to the students on techniques to use while caring for a pregnant woman (described in Chapter 5). During a break, some of the administrators began quietly talking about Carmelita and about how she was there not only to teach the students—but also to scope out the city as a possible new place to practice. Back in her own city up north, she had recently heard that another traditional midwife had been attacked, beaten, and robbed in her home because word had gotten out that she had many patients and therefore, possibly, was making good money. Carmelita had also begun to receive threatening phone calls, especially because of her own thriving midwifery practice. Violence was not something relegated to those involved in drug cartels; even elderly traditional midwives were becoming victims.

The escalation of drug-related murders and abductions, as well as the distrust in the government's tactics in a seemingly unbeatable "war" against drugs, contributed to a sense of pervasive fear and frustration. A background level of violence was becoming the norm (in Mexico and across Latin America), and people continued their daily lives, working around violence with different routes for travel, earlier curfews for their children, and redirected business ventures. Indeed, while finishing this book, I read with concern that the Mexican Midwifery Association had posted on their Facebook page a list of things their members should do or not do to avoid being robbed or kidnapped out of their cars as they drove to work (something that could be especially important for midwives, who often are called in the middle of the night). Each day new stories of the cartels' inventive techniques seemed to ratchet the threshold of violent possibilities up a notch. News of the ongoing femicides on the US–Mexico border was still a concern, sparking debate about women's safety more generally. Bus lines had developed separate buses for women only, just as metro services in Mexico City offered women-only cars during peak hours—both moves a reaction to fears of increasing violence against women. Everyone was exhausted by such violence, embarrassed by it on a national scale, and angry that nothing seemed to be improving. However, because of the confusion in many stories about who was more at fault—drug cartels or the government—people were wary to speak up or get involved for fear of becoming the next target.

The midwives involved in the campaign against obstetric violence drew on this national trope of violence in two distinct ways. First, they aligned themselves with current social concerns about specific kinds of violence that had come under increasing public scrutiny in order to argue for specific changes in obstetric care. Second, they sought to reveal patterns of structural violence which had allowed the persistence of outdated obstetric practices and which shaped provider attitudes toward women. In this first endeavor, pressing social concerns around escalating drug violence nationwide, femicides, and high rates of domestic violence were all evoked as a way to harness negative social and political attitudes toward violence in Mexico today. In the second endeavor, historical legacies of inequality based on gender, race, and class were revealed as ongoing concerns with direct impacts on women's bodies and health.

Perhaps the most powerful initiative of the obstetric violence movement was its attempt to link specific kinds of violence with the social structures that allow them to prevail. Obstetric violence, they argued, is not the product of rogue individual practitioners' acts but rather of a systemic failure that reinforces outdated practices. Whereas other forms of gendered violence, such as domestic violence—which has gained visibility as a widespread social concern in Mexico in recent years (Castro, Peek-Asa, and Ruiz 2003; Diaz Olavarrieta and Sotelo 1996)—continue to be framed in terms of actions like spousal abuse and intimate relationships, the campaign against obstetric violence aligned itself more with work that framed gendered issues within their historical and political contexts and which must be addressed publicly and regulated by the state. For example, Kaja Finkler (1994) argues that broad historical processes, pervasive cultural attitudes toward women, and the daily stresses women face in Mexico result in the patterns of sickness found there. Further, she argues that once women can "change their existence to allow a restoration of dignity within the society at large and within the confines of their homes," then we will see equal sickness rates between men and women (209). In order to address the tangible inequalities in health seen across gendered divisions, then, we must address these deeper cultural understandings.

This explicit emphasis on underlying structural inequalities, along with the strong language and legal repercussions outlined in the obstetric violence movement, contrast with the earlier and ongoing humanization of birth movement, which was more about individual choices and responsibilities. The midwives were making conscious choices to shift their focus from a grassroots movement to one that calls for accountability from the state at the highest levels. As the midwives from Nueve Lunas expressed, they hoped that the public would be moved by the discourse around obstetric violence and would begin to reframe their negative experiences with the health-care system in terms of violation and abuse, ultimately pressuring practitioners to change. However, the movement against obstetric violence offered a more nuanced critique of neoliberal health care in Mexico, which had put responsibilities for care onto the individual, and its goal focused on changing norms and regulatory procedures from the top down.

By not framing the obstetric violence movement as completely a people's movement steeped in grassroots activism, the midwives also revealed, on the one hand, sensitivity to the possible issues that could arise for women who would be asked to speak out against their care providers—a position that is not taken up easily or without consequence. Women were bound to certain kinds of health providers and clinics due to availability, or, at the time, by their association with the national conditional cash transfer system, IMSS Oportunidades, which paid them if they completed their prenatal and delivery care in a certified clinic. Many had signed on to the relatively new national free health insurance program, Seguro Popular, which also obliged them to see certain practitioners and to deliver in the program's hospitals. Thus, women may be stuck with certain providers and not have the resources or the authority to demand better care—a situation which the midwives were quick to point out stems from unequal racial, classist, and gendered relationships.

On the other hand, it was not purely altruistic sensitivity that drove the midwives' campaign against violence. Rather, this movement must be understood as a reflection of their increased presence in state institutions and their increasingly authoritative voice on women's health in Mexico.

Conclusion

Is there a way to talk about structural violence without recourse to metaphor or moral assumptions? Is there a way to talk about direct physical violence without obscuring underlying patterns of inequality? As Mexican midwives discussed obstetric violence, they attempted to hold structural violence alongside physical violence as equally problematic trends in the health-care system. Structural violence, they argued, motivates both the infrastructural failings described in Chapter 3—insufficient roads, radios, beds, etc.—and the mistreatment described here. In doing this, however, they ran the risk of alienating doctors and political allies by defining such violence too broadly. This could be counterproductive to the tentative partnership they had built with the health-care system.

On the other hand, two contextual processes were making it possible for the midwives' concerns to gain purchase—or at least to get attention. First, international pressures to lower maternal mortality had resulted in Mexico's investment in professional midwifery as a low-cost intervention (a process I discuss in Chapter 2). Thus, midwives were increasingly present in policy discussions and in public hospitals, where they rotated as students and later worked as professionals. In these roles, they worked with, within, and alongside the health-care system as allies and agents of its mission, and they thus had access and a place from which to voice their opinions. Second, national anxieties about widespread social violence had primed the public to react negatively to depictions of violence in spaces that were previously considered safe. The very pairing of the terms "obstetric" and "violence" is unexpected, jarring, and provocative. In a time when violence was seeping into people's homes, the notion that it exists in obstetrics may not have seemed as surprising.

What would it look like to eradicate obstetric violence? When I asked student midwives to envision their ideal conditions for birth, they drew pictures that offer some ideas of how they would answer that question. In Figure 8, the pregnant woman is saying, "Yes I have many pains, I want to take a bath and drink water." Her husband stands at her side, drawn smaller than she. To her other side are the midwife and two students, who are saying, "Yes, we will help her, she wants to eat," and "She breathes and wants to walk." The scene takes place outside, but there is also an indoor room drawn, with a bed, television, and bathtub. In general, students drew pictures in which women had agency and choice. Figure 9, for example, shows a woman laboring vertically, holding onto a rope for counter pressure; a birthing tub sits as an option in front of her. Her husband supports her from behind, while the midwife (indicated as the artist herself) watches from the corner. Many drawings also showed women in outdoor spaces with natural elements around them. Another important theme was happiness: drawings with midwives showed smiling women, smiling midwives, and often smiling babies as well. These kinds of scenes did not always reflect the reality of the births students were seeing, but they highlight what students saw as the missing elements in quality care.

For the midwives in this study, legislating and policing hospital norms of best practices in obstetrics was just the beginning of the path to creating the conditions for the kinds of births they wanted to see in their country. Even as the midwives continue to struggle to determine the appropriate ways to humanize obstetrics through outlawing certain practices—like manual uterine revisions or the insertion of IUDs immediately postpartum—they confront the impossibility of changing institutional and provider attitudes toward patients. "What was I supposed to do," asked one midwifery student rhetorically when describing a hospital birth she had recently observed, "when the doctor threw his tape measure in the patient's face when she complained in labor? He just hated her, for no reason. I could not do anything to help her."

I do not suggest that all women are treated in this way in Mexican public hospitals; during my research many physicians were backing the movement to combat obstetric violence, alongside midwives and other activists. Often, the doctors expressed the violence most articulately, as they found themselves entrenched in systems where inherited protocols dictated how women were treated and what doctors were supposed to do. For the midwives, who are suddenly being thrust into a medical system that has marginalized midwifery for decades, the violence they encounter stands in overt contrast to the humanized model that midwifery champions. It also stands in contrast to the goals of global health initiatives that seek to improve health outcomes through a commitment to evidence-based practices in medicine. Obstetric violence is violent not just because of the pain it can cause women but also because it does not lead to better, safer, healthier patients.

This is perhaps the point by which midwives will gain the most traction in their push to recognize and regulate obstetric violence. The midwives

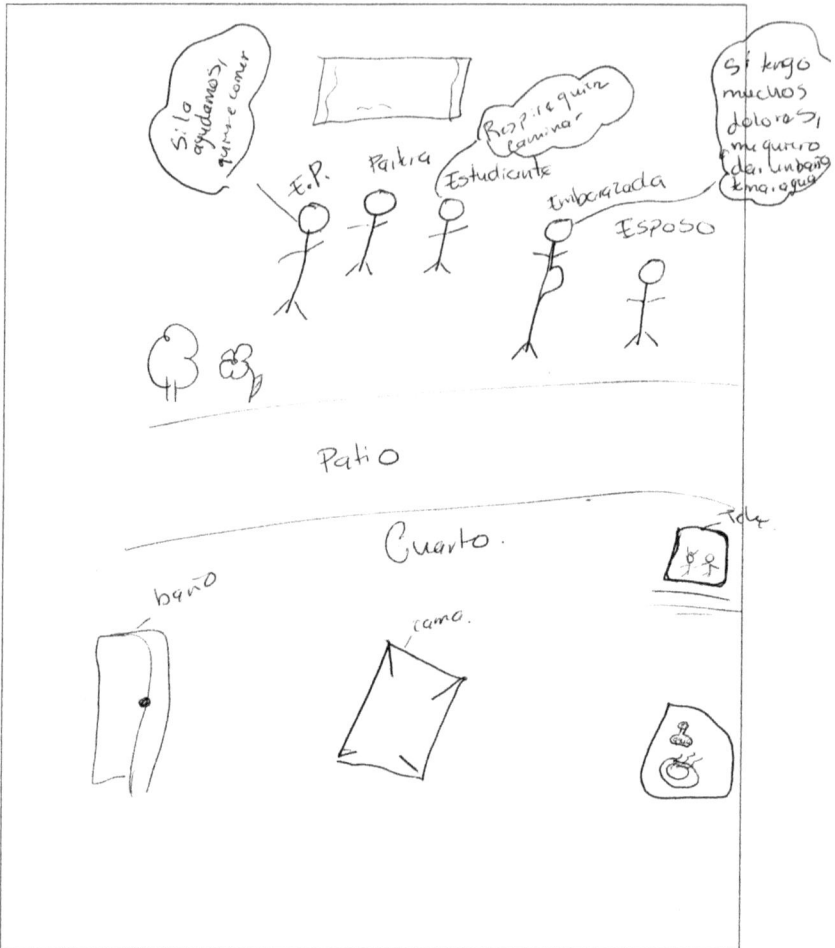

FIGURE 8: A midwifery student's drawing of how an ideal birth should look, depicted on the patio of a home with family and midwives.

have internalized the message that, as Nadine said, "Mexico doesn't actually care about women." So, if they are going to change the way birth is managed in Mexico, they have to show why violence against women is bad for health outcomes and, ultimately, bad for the country. In this way, as in so many others, midwives are pragmatic.

They are pragmatic as they continue to resist a complete shift to biomedical practices and institutions because, aside from the infrastructural and gender-based violence they find within them, they recognize that those practices and institutions are not always what women need or are even able

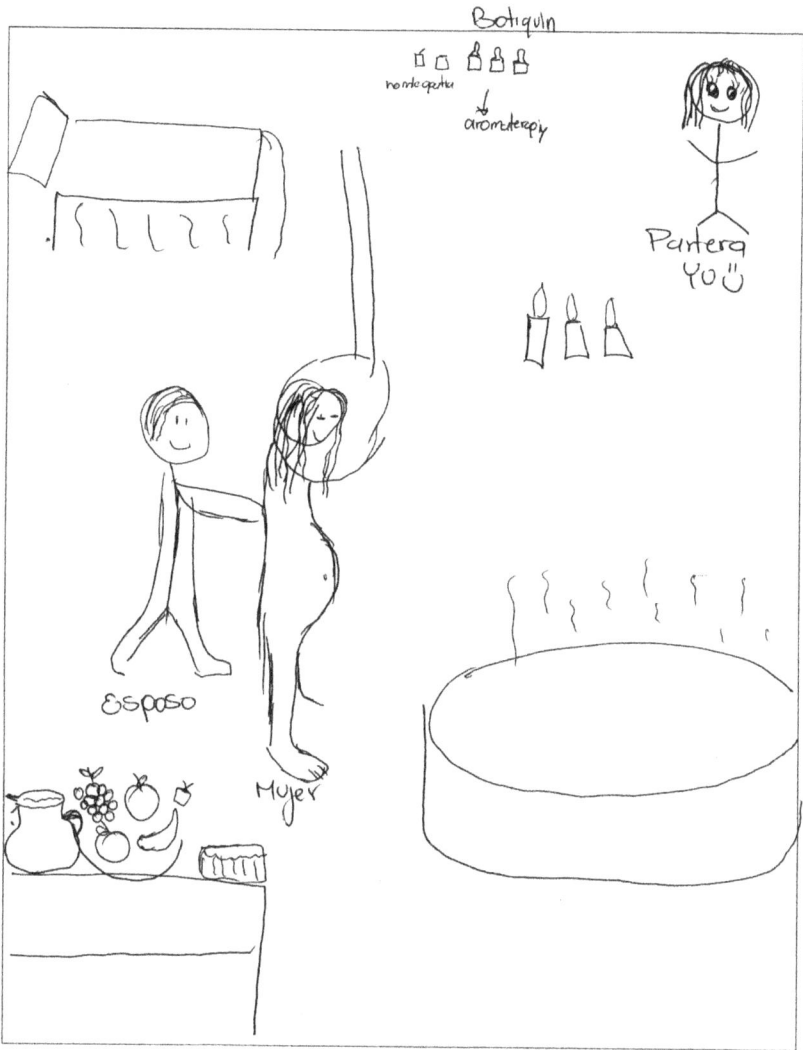

FIGURE 9: A midwifery student's drawing of an ideal birth setting, including a vertical birth rope and bathtub.

to access. As midwives attend diverse women across Mexico, they draw strategically on a set of practices, technologies, treatments, and ideologies that have roots outside biomedicine and that I refer to as the contemporary version of "traditional midwifery." Why traditional midwifery persists and how it continues to make sense within the context of a rapidly medicalized setting for birth in Mexico is the focus of the next chapter.

CHAPTER 5

Modern Tradition

Throughout this book, I have written about the many ways midwives in Mexico tried to create routes to professional careers, standardize relationships with the health and education systems, and institutionalize midwifery's approach to holistic, humanistic care. But not all midwives had access to institutionalized educational programs like CASA or Mujeres Aliadas (discussed in previous chapters), and not all midwives thought that midwifery should have to achieve formal state recognition. Indeed, for many midwives and many families, the idea of "professional midwifery" sounded too medical or too far from what they saw as the roots of midwifery as a traditional, locally based practice. While CASA and Mujeres Aliadas schools integrated traditional Mexican midwifery practices (along with alternative practices from around the world) into their curricula, they saw them as complementary and secondary to a core body of knowledge based in biomedical education.

Despite its marginalized position within the official curricula, however, nearly all of the midwifery students told me how important traditional midwifery was to them. Further, as I traveled around Mexico, spoke with midwives of diverse backgrounds, and spent time at midwifery gatherings, I saw that the role of the traditional midwife continued to be seen as valid and valuable to practitioners as well, albeit to varying degrees. This finding did not fully align with what the numbers said—that traditional midwives were fading out[1]—or what some of the professional midwifery school administrators and politicians were saying—that the best way forward was one that worked with the health-care system and was based to some degree on a biomedical model.

In this chapter, I ask: why does traditional midwifery persist? I ask this while recognizing that the numbers of those who consider themselves traditional midwives are dwindling, and that midwifery as a whole is indeed changing. I also ask this while recognizing that there are facets of traditional midwifery—and traditional medicine more broadly—that have become trendy and appeal to those who can pay when others are stuck going to the public hospital for economic reasons (that is, if those facets are not institutionalized or widely available within free or low-cost settings) (Vega 2018). I ask this because I heard midwives and their students tell me again and again how important it was to them to protect, learn, and pass on the knowledge of their predecessors.

I take traditional midwifery here as a flexible idea because it is the only manner I know of how to talk about the various ways I saw it described and employed. After years of taking note of when, where, and how traditional midwifery was evoked, I came to this conclusion: traditional midwifery encompasses a fluid set of practices, technologies, treatments, and ideologies that have roots outside the structures of biomedical health-care training and services (though, as many anthropologists have shown, often find their way into biomedical settings. See, for example, Langwick 2008; Zhan 2009). I call these "fluid" because it is important to recognize up front that these practices, technologies, treatments, and ideologies are not static remnants of Mexico's past but rather emerge from interactions between practitioners and change over time. As such, traditional midwifery can encompass the CASA-educated, professional midwives whose mantra is to go to natural remedies first and seek biomedical remedies as a last resort. It also encompasses the practitioners like Juana (written about in my Introduction) who apprenticed to become a village midwife but had picked up technologies and treatments from biomedical training programs over the years. Traditional midwifery, like professional midwifery, draws from multiple sources and changes over time (this is not to say that all exchanges are equal but rather that which we deem "traditional" has always been in flux).

Traditional midwifery was woven through all the spaces I spent time in during fieldwork, in ways that, as an ethnographer, I would sometimes see full force and sometimes just catch a glimpse of. I began to pay attention to what traditional midwifery meant to the people who talked about it, employed it, and defended it. I saw that there was urgency behind their desire for it to continue, this evolving blend of elements that "count" as traditional midwifery. This urgency and the schools, practitioners, and conferences that build on it are the engines behind traditional midwifery's persistence. But how do we explain this persistence, given the forward momentum of biomedical expansion, the tendency to tokenize traditional practices and practitioners, and the global health push to universalize training models and approaches to care?

Three things emerged from my data that explain this persistence. The first is that traditional midwifery is inherently a political idea: in its very name is the idea that it existed *prior* to colonialism and the universalizing principles of global health and biomedicine. In their many proclamations that we need to "preserve and protect" traditional midwifery, midwives were calling for a revaluation of the knowledge that had long been stripped away or devalued by the encroachment of Western practices, technologies, and ideologies. In this way, efforts to teach and practice traditional midwifery are subversive. They have brought attention to the ways in which what was known in Mexico had long been devalued and seen as, in the best light, less than adequate and, in the worst, dangerous. In a related way, traditional midwifery is political because it is tied to a revaluation of women's bodies and choices: providing women the right to choose practitioners or practices that make them feel respected or comforted pushes back against hegemonic biomedical institutions that have long told women what they have to do and how they have to do it when it comes to their bodies and reproduction.

The second explanation is that traditional midwifery is pragmatic, not dogmatic. I saw again and again how midwives would weigh the needs of their patients, the tools at hand, and their own knowledge before deciding which kinds of tools to reach for: the electronic Doppler or the no-tech fetoscope, the tincture or the prescription pad, the massage or the referral to the public hospital. These tools, technologies, and treatments were not only from ancestral Mexican origins; midwives drew liberally from an array of worldly alternative approaches that they categorized as traditional (such as homeopathic medicines from Germany; flower essences, developed in their modern form in England; or acupressure from China). Many practitioners felt strongly opposed to any biomedical treatments (they would often refer to them as a last resort), but none would hesitate to refer a woman they deemed in crisis to the hospital or deny someone an antibiotic for an infection. In this way, they were trying to show that traditional midwifery could coexist with biomedical backup when necessary. What sometimes smacked of dogmatism to those who saw traditional midwifery proponents as anti-biomedicine was, I argue, not a reflection of midwives insisting that their way was the only way but rather the necessary stance of those fighting to uphold their value when it is systematically being taken from them.

Finally, traditional midwifery is itself modern. It treats modern bodies experiencing problems brought on by modern life. In this way it is not about a return to a romanticized past. The past is, as I said above, valued and respected through the use of the term "traditional," and many traditional midwives do use remedies or techniques that have been in circulation for centuries (such as the use of the Mexican shawl called the *rebozo*); however, when traditional midwifery is seen as merely a remnant of a Mexican past, the contemporary issues that midwives reveal and treat become obscured. I argue that we must not gloss over traditional midwives' approaches as outdated or quaint but rather interrogate what they can tell us about what contemporary women need and want and how these practitioners fill those needs.

The ethnographic stories in this chapter illustrate these arguments within a range of settings where traditional midwifery persists. I first describe a series of scenes from an international midwifery conference in San Cristobal de las Casas, Chiapas, then trace the details of one prenatal visit with a professional midwife at CASA in San Miguel de Allende, Guanajuato, and finally end on a discussion of the complexities involved in the design of Nueve Lunas traditional midwifery school in Oaxaca City, Oaxaca.

This chapter also shows how traditional midwifery is changing and must be viewed as a dynamic profession that exists in the modern world rather than as an ancestral remnant of Mexico's past. I show how traditional midwifery is changed as it passes from one midwife to another, how it changes in interactions with formal and informal educational processes, and how its champions are trying to design flexible models of traditional training so that even as it changes, it is not lost.

What Does "Traditional" Midwifery Mean?

Traditional midwives and their practices have been the focus of much anthropological writing, especially since the publication of Brigitte Jordan's classic ethnography, *Birth in Four Cultures*, in 1978. In the decades following Jordan's book, studies have examined alternatives to biomedical approaches to women's health care across global contexts and from varying angles, describing the overlapping categories of traditional midwives, empirical midwives, traditional birth attendants, and Indigenous birth attendants. Within these studies, alternative birth practices and their practitioners have been framed in different ways: as connections to local traditional histories, as revolutionary practitioners, as targets of biomedical colonization, and as a form of resistance against the hegemonic biomedical institution by seeking to return power to women (Simonds, Rothman, and Norman 2006).

Proponents of traditional Mexican midwifery refer consistently to the intimate relationship between traditional midwives and their cultural contexts; within anthropology this relationship has also been stressed. Cecilia Benoit and Robbie Davis-Floyd argue that "neither midwives' knowledge base nor their socialization are arbitrary; rather, each is shaped by the larger culture and structure of society that generates it" (Benoit and Davis-Floyd 2004, 183). This is not to say that traditional practitioners are confined by their immediate geographical boundaries; rather, the manifestations of information flowing throughout space and across time become evident in practitioners' notions of tradition. Similarly, Mei Zhan has illuminated how traditional healing practices in general must be understood as co-created through the multiple entanglements they have with "translocal encounters and from discrepant locations." For Zhan, traditional practices are "made *through*—rather than prior to" these encounters (2009, 1).

By situating traditional midwifery within social and political systems, anthropologists have argued that it is important to avoid romanticizing midwifery as an a-historical phenomenon that stands outside current manifestations of inequality. Rather, we must consider traditional midwives and their practices as current reflections of modern power and resistance. Midwives in Bijnor, India, for example, are seen not as possessors of special knowledge or skills but rather as women of equally low status as the other women in their social class (Jeffery and Jeffery 1993). Such observations are important because they challenge the trope of the midwife as a revered alternative to colonizing biomedicine and urge us to contextualize midwives instead within their actual social context. Patricia Kaufert and John O'Neil (1993) further argue that we must understand midwifery as belonging to a fluid category that is directly affected by the political economy in which they work. Midwives in the Inuit Canadian northwest, for example, have been devalued as an effect of the government's push to have women give birth in hospitals. What a midwife stands for in her social and historical context cannot be assumed as stable or universal; I look here, then, at the specific case of traditional midwives in Mexico in order to both understand and problematize their representation.

Anthropologists have also critiqued an assumed division between traditional midwives and their biomedical counterparts, although often their studies begin with this very dichotomy. Faye Ginsburg and Rayna Rapp point out that "much of the research on Indigenous birth attendants originates in evaluations of biomedical interventions" (1991, 322). In such work, alternative birthing practices highlight concerns about biomedicine's practices and rapid expansion into developing countries. Nuanced studies of the relationship between biomedical and alternative birthing practices are not one-dimensional, however. Rather, they reveal that "midwives may both appropriate and resist the centralizing, professionalizing tendencies of clinically based birth in their geographic area" (1991, 322). It has become more broadly understood within anthropology that traditional medicine does not exist as a separate entity from biomedicine but rather that the two are complicit and intertwined (Langwick 2011). Mexico's traditional midwives are inevitably entangled with biomedicine's reach, whether they embrace it to some extent or reject it wholeheartedly.

Indeed, it became clear to me quickly during my fieldwork that the term "traditional midwifery" was complicated even within the midwifery community, as it had a history of being reimagined by Mexican public health efforts over the years in ways that changed what it meant to practice traditional midwifery. Fernanda, then director of the CASA professional midwifery program, told me in 2010 that "proponents of traditional midwifery do not realize that many of the things being practiced by these traditional midwives are either dangerous or are not 'traditional' at all!" She went on to explain that many of the techniques being used by traditional midwives are a result of government interventions begun in the early twentieth century, at which time the government began rounding up the traditional midwives and training them in brief workshops designed to teach them basic obstetric skills and emergency responses (see El Kotni 2019 for a history of these trainings). Midwives recalled how they used to sell pre-loaded syringes of Pitocin in Mexican pharmacies and that traditional midwives were taught in their trainings to use it preemptively during labor but without much guidance as to dosage or timing.[2] This resulted in some midwives injecting women repeatedly until the uterus would get so hard that they could not get the baby out, leading to maternal and fetal deaths. Eventually, "all this training molded the 'traditional' midwifery of Mexico into something that now has little to do with tradition," exclaimed Fernanda.

Fernanda's concerns were not expressed to me as a way of denigrating the practices of traditional midwives, who she seemed to genuinely respect. Instead, her point was that discussions about what traditional midwives know and do must be informed by an awareness of how they have changed and of the historical influences of state interventions. She felt it important that advocates of traditional midwives' rights did not gloss over this history, though she also had real concerns about the potential impacts of such interventions. These concerns motivated her passion for midwifery education on its own terms.

Yet, as I found throughout my research, many traditional midwives and their supporters continued to depict traditional midwifery as ancient, locally specific, and individualized, despite documented and often problematic interconnections with biomedical trainings. Margaret MacDonald's (2007) work on Canadian midwifery reveals that this kind of framing can be a double-edged sword. In Canada, she argues, the depiction of midwifery as an ancient, traditional craft—one which stands in opposition to biomedicine—has done two different things: on the one hand, such depictions "have been symbolically important and politically strategic for practitioners, users, and advocates of midwifery," while on the other hand they have "been identified as the source of midwifery's lack of legitimacy by those who oppose it." MacDonald concludes that "midwifery in Canada has not been reclaimed or resurrected from the past so much as it has been reinvented in the present, out of present-day concerns," such that it "is a product of local social and historical specificity, imaginative connections with ideas of universality, and international midwifery networks and knowledge exchange" (2007, 7). Traditional Mexican midwives and their supporters understand and navigate these networks, yet continue to present traditional knowledge as something that exists outside them. For these midwives, traditional knowledge cannot be separated from traditional ways of knowing, which are, to them, inherently individualized and local.

Saber Nacer: Who Knows How to Be Born?

Even as schools were incorporating elements of traditional midwifery into their curricula (such as through CASA's yearly home stays with traditional midwives or guest speakers teaching about herbs at Mujeres Aliadas), there was a common sentiment that the ultimate trajectory of traditional knowledge came through ancestral ties. Midwifery is, after all, an ancient profession; for those who practiced traditional midwifery, paying respect to ancestral midwives and explicitly linking their knowledge to their foremothers was important to them. In this way, traditional midwifery knowledge is personal and intimate—it comes through ties to other women, often family or close relations in the community.

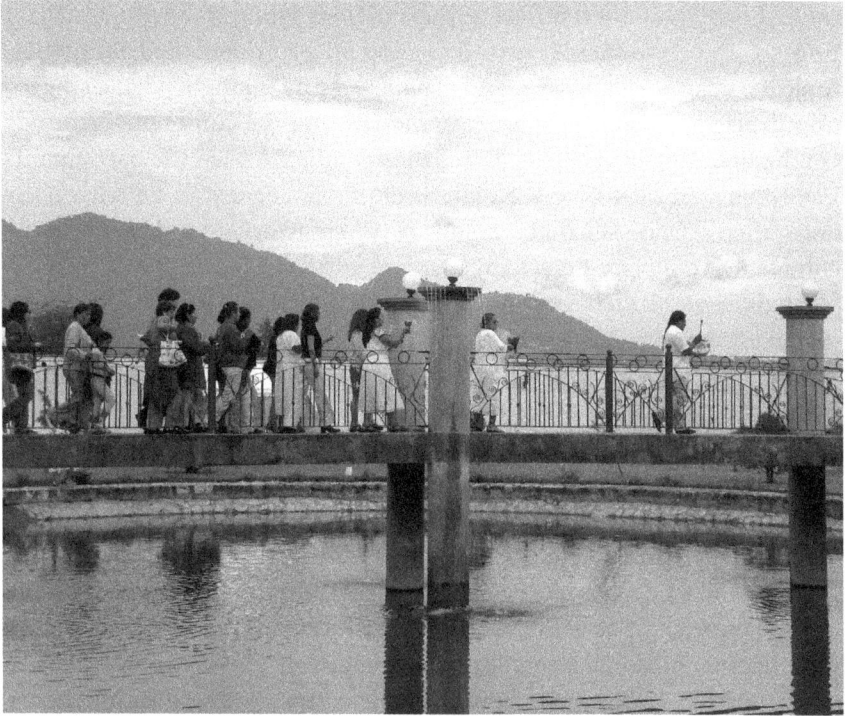

FIGURE 10: Opening ceremony at Saber Nacer midwifery conference in San Cristobal de las Casas, Chiapas, 2010. Photo by author.

In the summer of 2010 I attended an international conference on midwifery in San Cristobal de las Casas, Chiapas, called Saber Nacer (To Know How to be Born). Organized by the Luna Maya (Maya Moon) midwifery clinic and training site in the same city, it had been advertised as a conference meant to bring together midwives and birth workers from across Mexico—and beyond—to discuss and learn about diverse techniques and issues in women's reproductive health. In attendance at this conference were traditional and professional midwifery students and teachers from across Mexico, Mexican public health investigators, European practitioners, leaders of midwifery organizations, and publications from the United States and Canada. Most noticeably, there were perhaps fifty traditional midwives who had been bussed in from around Mexico and Guatemala, separated into groups by dialect, region, and clothing style. The conference was supposed to be a space for an equal exchange of ideas and techniques among traditional, professional, and international groups of midwives, yet the program's set-ting, style, and emphases were all focused on traditional (and alternative) midwifery skills, treatments, and products. More than 450 people showed up, surprising even the organizers and packing the conference grounds. On the first morning, the local traditional midwives led the participants in a ceremony; blessings were said over plants laid out in a circle on the grass, then a procession led everyone over a small bridge and back into the conference room (see Figure 10).

Attendees took their seats and faced the stage. "Saber Nacer is a reminder that women and babies know how to birth. Nature has created an elegant system that gives wisdom to women and babies. This knowledge is built in to women and babies, bodies and blood. Midwives are the guardians of this knowledge," began the speaker who opened the conference. She was from the United States—the president of a large North American midwifery organization—and spoke in English. She spoke firmly but slowly, and in the dramatic pauses between her statements, translations into Spanish and regional languages like Tzotzil could be heard rippling across the large conference space. The words took a while to be translated, but the message was clear—traditional midwifery knowledge was personal and linked to one's connections to nature, bodies, and ancestry. To drive the point home, the speaker brought a few colleagues onto the stage and had them lead a sing-along, chanting a cappella: "We are drownin' out the rhythm on our ancestors' feet." Eventually, everyone was standing and singing, though in the cacophony, the meaning was less tied to the words and more to the collective effort. As people stamped and sang, they looked around and smiled at each other.

The idea that traditional knowledge was personal and passed down through ancestral ties was repeated throughout my fieldwork and indeed was emphasized throughout the Saber Nacer conference. This was knowl-edge that midwives felt could not be taught in schools (or at least, not only in schools). During lunch that day, I sat next to an older traditional midwife from a nearby mountain community who explained how knowledge came to her as a midwife. She was all smiles, the metal caps covering all of her front teeth shining as she recounted stories about some of the nearly two hundred births that she had attended over the course of her career. "How did you learn to be a midwife?" I asked her, conversationally. She told me about dreams that she began to have when she was younger, in which an old ancestor would explain to her differences between plants that could be useful for medicinal healing. "She would tell me, 'This plant to prevent hemorrhage, but be sure it has purple flowers, not the white ones.' And then I found it, growing by the river, and we still use that plant!" After she had become known in her community for having knowledge about plants, she was called one day to her first birth. "I had no real training, I just went because everyone thought that the woman and her baby would die. But I received wisdom from God—he told me to heat the towels, to use *manzanilla* (chamomile)—and in the end, the baby was fine," she recounted. It is possible that this midwife had learned from others in her community about midwifery and plants, yet what interests me is how she herself frames her entrance into midwifery. In her story, training came from a spiritual connection and through the community's decision to call on her as the most authoritative knowledge on plants and healing.

Violeta, another traditional midwife who spoke at the conference, repeated this notion of being called by the community and of inheriting knowledge. "The first time I delivered a baby alone, I was fourteen years old," Violeta told one group of assembled midwifery students.

> My mother was a midwife, but no one else was home, and a man arrived at my house telling me I had to go with him to help his wife, who was in labor. I went, and everything was going fine, until the woman was about to deliver her placenta. Suddenly, I noticed that it did not look right—it was in fact not the placenta, but another baby. My first birth as a midwife, I was all alone and delivered *twins*! My mother got home later and was angry at me for doing this by myself, but I didn't have a choice!

Violeta described how her own children now accompany her and learn from her, a process that she said is "like a tradition now." Thus, tradition here takes on the double meaning of a form of knowledge that is differentiated from science and a way of learning that happens between mothers and their children. This second meaning of tradition is important because it links this category of knowledge to a particular social and historical context. Knowledge that is passed between women is not dependent on formal structures of education. In a country where nearly 5 percent of the population is illiterate, most illiteracy is concentrated in Indigenous, rural areas, and more than half of the illiterate are women, the traditional role of handing down knowledge via other routes cannot be discounted (Narro Robles and Moctezuma Navarro 2012).

Another common way that traditional midwives described how they learned was through a differentiation from science-based education. Violeta was quick to note to the students that "I have no scientific knowledge; I cannot say that I learned from a book. I learned *traditional* knowledge, and that is what I use when I give consultations in my home." This comment served both as a proud marker of Violeta's lineage and as a justification, perhaps, for any gaps in her "scientific" knowledge. Similarly, Doña Guadalupe, one of the founders of CASA's midwifery school who still teaches and sees patients there, consistently introduces herself in conferences and meetings by reminding everyone that "*Yo soy partera tradicional,* no *profesional*" (I am a traditional midwife, *not* a professional one). By distinguishing herself as traditional, and not professional, Doña Guadalupe marks her way of knowing (and, in her job, teaching) as distinct from professional knowledge.

Traditional midwifery knowledge is not only passed through generations of women; there exist both casual flows of knowledge between friends and colleagues as well as structured moments of teaching in which traditional midwives impart their knowledge through midwife-organized trainings, workshops, or conferences. These latter modes of transmission are becoming increasingly the primary ways that traditional midwifery knowledge gets passed on to others, as traditional midwives are aging and dying out, and younger women in their communities are less interested in learning from them and carrying on the midwifery career. Traditional midwives who continue to practice also use these methods to network with each other, especially if they do not have other local, practicing traditional midwives with whom to discuss techniques or tools. However, many traditional midwives I spoke to agreed that conferences often turned out to be performative spectacles or social occasions. Often, the conferences were put on with too much foreign influence or with foreign attendees in mind. One traditional midwife told me that when she announced to her colleagues that she wanted to get registered with the state as an "official" traditional midwife, "they told me that I had better learn English so that foreigners could come take me to conferences."

Doña Guadalupe, for example, admitted to me at the Saber Nacer conference that she much preferred to learn from individual midwives rather than through such large conferences. She said that the conference itself was a political and social experience, not a place where you could really pick up new skills. Her method of learning, she said, was to directly ask traditional midwives wherever she travels (and she travels often, due to her position as one of CASA's founders) about what kinds of plants are available in their regions for certain pregnancy or labor concerns. I had seen her prescribe leaves from the plant *zoapatle* as a natural oxytocic alternative to the drug Pitocin, used to bring on contractions in many patients who had passed their due dates and needed to be nudged into labor. She kept a plastic grocery bag of the dull green leaves in her desk drawer so that she could offer a handful to a patient when necessary, instructing them to brew a strong tea with the leaves and wait to see if labor ensued. When she traveled, she said, she was always interested in what other traditional midwives used to induce labor or speed things along. "Here in this region, we use the *zoapatle*, but the name varies in different regions. When I was traveling in the South, in Chiapas, I asked them what herb they used there, and they told me about a different one, called *puntitia del níspero*, which turned out to be the young leaves of the *níspero* (loquat) plant." In these person-to-person interactions, knowledge passes between traditional midwives; it is local knowledge, passed on an individual basis, not through books or databases. In many cases, it is not applicable across geographical boundaries—some plants only grow in some regions, and thus midwives find their own local variations. Books do exist, although it would seem that they are considered to be mostly for professional midwives, researchers, or other interested outsiders—anthropologists, perhaps?—who want to learn about traditional medicine. For example, one book that was being passed around in the midwifery school in Oaxaca had been written by Doña Queta, a traditional midwife from nearby who was known for her knowledge of medicinal plants. The book, entitled *Medicina tradicional: Doña Queta y el legado de los habitantes de las nubes* (Guerra Falcon 2009; Traditional medicine: Doña Queta and the legend of the cloud dwellers), had nice big color photographs and was making the rounds of midwifery conferences around the country. The prohibitively high price tag—six hundred Mexican pesos, or about forty-five US dollars at the time—made it clear that this was not necessarily meant as a traditional midwives' desk reference but rather an anthropological collector's item.

In a country where women—especially rural and Indigenous women—have historically had less access to formal education (as discussed in Chapter 1), individual apprenticeships and self-reliance make sense. As education rates improve, however, many traditional midwives worry that the next generation will not want to carry on their ways of knowing. Their daughters wanted to move to larger cities, and if they were interested in their mothers' career paths, they opted to study nursing or medicine. At stake for the existing traditional midwives is not only the loss of traditional midwifery but also the loss of a way of knowing that is based on their personal connections to other midwives—primarily female relatives. Further at stake is the loss of ingenuity that is integral to traditional midwifery. That is, what many traditional midwives came to share in the Saber Nacer conference were techniques for dealing with complications in labor that they had found ways to resolve because there was no one else to help. The lowest education levels in Mexico map onto the places that most lack access to biomedical care, and thus traditional ways of knowing have filled in the gap to provide the kinds of care necessary for the particular needs of their communities. Their practices were being shaped by pragmatism: they were doing what needed to be done because there was often not another choice.

"¡O pares . . . o pares!": Pragmatism and Practice

I began thinking about the connection between pragmatism and practice as I reflected on the second afternoon of the Saber Nacer conference, when I had ducked out of a sudden onset of pouring rain and into one of the smaller buildings being used to house some of the midwives who could not afford a hotel. I found a spot to sit on a futon in the corner and nursed my third cup of tea of the day, marveling over the coziness of this space, the constantly full teakettle, the tray of chocolates—all details provided to make attendees feel comfortable. As I settled in to warm up, I noticed that there was an intense conversation going on just on the next futon. An elder traditional midwife, speaking Tzotzil and being translated into Spanish by her younger companion, was talking to a group of young midwives held in rapt attention. She was telling them how she delivers breech babies (babies who are born in a seated position, instead of head-first). "You hold the bottom and pull gently during contractions," she told them, her hands moving in front of her as if holding a baby. "Rotate as you go, back and forth . . . the head may be stuck for up to fifteen minutes." The students leaned closer—delivering a breech baby is considered dangerous and high risk, the kind of thing that traditional midwives are supposed to refer to physicians. On their faces, I could see the fear, mixed with awe, as they pictured the baby with its head stuck for a full quarter of an hour. The traditional midwife went on to resolve the tension by saying that if the baby *did* end up coming out "pale and lifeless," you should put the placenta into the fire, or even just in hot water, and this would make the life come back into the baby. The students took in the advice, nodding seriously.

The skills presented in stories like this serve an important purpose, I suggest: to highlight other possible ways of knowing and other possible practices, all in contrast to biomedical options. Not only do they stand in contrast to science, however, but also to the access to modernity and urban resources that have been tied to it. Breech baby? No problem. Lifeless newborn? Just heat up the placenta. These stories serve as an important reminder to midwives—who may be working in rural, isolated areas where they are the only care providers—that there are always things you can do, even if you do not have the latest in technology or medicine. As the traditional midwife, Violeta, pointed out, "In the communities, everyone knows you won't be having a cesarean section or anything like that. *¡O pares . . . o pares!*" (Either you give birth . . . or you give birth!).

The sharing of birth stories, especially difficult births that get resolved by the midwife's ingenuity, builds confidence and trust into the community, both in their own abilities and in the birth process itself. The structure of the Mexican health-care system is such that scientific medical expertise flows from the urban centers outward, yet it doesn't always arrive in rural communities with any force, if it arrives at all. Midwives tell these stories of heroic action in the face of vast deficiencies in health-care resources, then, to mark the gaps that they find themselves filling. Interestingly, Violeta's assertion echoed the derogatory phrase I described in Chapter 1 that an obstetrician reminded CASA students about, as a way to alert them to public perceptions about midwifery: "The baby will come out with the midwife, without the midwife, or in spite of the midwife." The connotation is that midwives don't do anything to actually help during labor and birth and that ultimately the baby will be born one way or another. While this phrase demeans midwives' role as caregivers, Violeta's point about the inevitability of birth is that women in rural areas don't have the biomedical backup, and thus traditional midwives provide the only support.

This message was repeated when, later in the same day at the conference, I attended a session, led by a woman who identified herself as a traditional Maya midwife, on Maya abdominal massage during pregnancy. Commonly referred to as *sobada*, the massage is a technique used by traditional midwives to turn babies in utero by massaging the pregnant woman's abdomen and gently pushing the baby into position. I had to squeeze into a seat, because the room was packed full of women taking photographs and notes, as the presentation had already begun. The midwife was short, square, and around sixty years old, her long braid hanging like a thick rope down her back. She addressed the crowd from the front of the room, explaining that abdominal massage is a very versatile treatment, which can be used for all kinds of things that allopathic medicine cannot fix—she listed infertility, incontinence, ovarian cysts, pain with sex, endometriosis, lower back pain, and a poorly positioned baby as some of the possible symptoms that this procedure alleviates. She then gave us this story to illustrate the use of her massage:

> A woman showed up in pain, in labor, but the baby was trying to get out sideways. I began slowly massaging the baby during contractions to get it turned. The woman herself had the intuition to move her hips and sway around, and in the next contraction the baby came . . . the baby was dark blue and not breathing. But then I took the phlegm out of its mouth and began massaging the whole baby, and finally it began to cry. Then I blew on the baby lightly. Now, that baby is grown up.

As with the above story of the breech baby, this vignette carried its audience through a quick arc, climaxing in a moment of uncertainty and fear but resolving through the midwife's knowledge and skills.

With an attentive audience, the midwife continued by teaching them more about how Maya abdominal massage works to help women. When treating a non-pregnant patient, she explained, the massage has to do with the uterus and its position; if the uterus is not properly aligned, the body will not be in equilibrium, causing all sorts of problems. A uterus can fall for many reasons, she said; from a car accident, giving birth, or even wearing high heels. On pregnant women, the massage is mostly used to reposition the baby so that it is head down and ready for an easier delivery. She pointed to a visibly pregnant woman in the audience and asked if she would volunteer to have her baby turned for the group. The woman happily made her way to the front of the room and lay down on a long wooden table. The midwife felt her abdomen, nodding as she went, then announced that the baby was indeed upside down (with its head up). The audience leaned forward in their seats.

The midwife began to massage the woman's belly, rocking it back and forth and then slowly but firmly pushing the baby so that it would turn. After a few minutes of this, she felt for the baby's head near the woman's pubic bone. Then, taking a step back, she proclaimed the baby now head down. Camera flashes fired nonstop as the audience members angled to get better views of this demonstration. After a moment, the woman got up, smiling, and went to take her seat. People had lots of questions and especially wanted to know why she did that without checking the heart rate, at least, to make sure that the baby was not in stress or getting the umbilical cord wrapped around its neck. The midwife said that in her community, this is not a big deal—women get their babies turned through the pregnancy to make sure that the baby is head down when it comes to term. And anyway, she said, she can feel the baby's head and then feel for the cord to see if it is pulsating or around the baby's neck. That is how she knows that the baby is ok; why would she need to monitor its heart rate with additional technologies? Violeta, who had been sitting in the front row of this demonstration, stood up at this point, faced the audience, and reminded everyone that "we must understand the context; again, these are rural midwives living in isolated places far from hospital support." The crowd murmured their understanding, heads nodding. Violeta said that mothers want to know that the baby will be head down when labor starts so as to prevent a trip to the hospital should the baby be in the wrong position, so the idea of routinely pushing the baby into place throughout pregnancy makes sense to them.

In this context, the idea of pushing the baby into place—called "external cephalic version" in biomedical terminology—makes sense to mothers and midwives. When there is no backup emergency care within easy distance from where you live, you want to do everything possible to prevent complications. Yet this is not quite the same as the notion of preventative care under a biomedical model; traditional midwives are not necessarily sending women into town to get lab work done, screening them for gestational diabetes or even high blood pressure—both normal preventative diagnostics conducted in a biomedical setting. For these midwives, and the women they treat, preventative care revolves not around knowing the body through lab tests and mechanical tools but rather through listening to the woman and feeling the baby. Repetitive turning of the baby may not make sense as preventative care under a biomedical framework—it is not necessary that the baby be head down throughout the whole pregnancy—but when taken within the context of the kinds of risks these midwives strive to avoid, it makes more sense. As Alison Bastien, a teacher who worked with and has written about both professional and traditional midwifery students across Mexico (see, for example, Bastien 2019), told me, "These kinds of practices, they are a form of 'defensive medicine.'" By "defensive medicine," Bastien did not mean the kinds of over-prescribing or use of unnecessary procedures that doctors in the global north use to avoid lawsuits in their practices; she referenced a defensiveness not driven by litigious concerns. By employing traditional techniques to preemptively avoid potential future complications, midwives were acting in the best interests of their patients, given the conditions and their understanding of worst-case scenarios.

Even as fewer and fewer women have traditional midwives attend their births, they continue to visit them for these uterine massages throughout pregnancy, a phenomenon leading some of the midwives I interviewed to comment that traditional midwives across Mexico are reduced to being seen as *masajistas* (massage therapists). Yet, as I argued in previous chapters, midwifery is not (only) about assisting women in giving birth—it is a profession that is engaged with helping women throughout their reproductive lives and which is embedded in the diverse conditions in which their patients and communities live. In this way, traditional midwifery resists the kind of universalization or standardization that global health policies seek to enforce.

The push to standardize professional midwifery in Mexico is part of a global movement to combat maternal mortality by investing in new strategies that target the most at-risk populations. However, proponents of traditional midwifery argue and demonstrate that traditional midwifery is valuable because of its ability to respond most appropriately to the needs of individual communities—not because of any claims to universality. Standardized, biomedicalized forms of care that import ways of knowing from afar may not understand, respect, or approach local concerns to the same extent. Beyond the diverse needs of women in diverse contexts that traditional midwifery responds to, the very ways of knowing in traditional midwifery are shaped by local necessity—a reality that is not unique to nonbiomedical practitioners. Anthropologists have long illustrated the ways that practitioners' knowledge is shaped by the circumstances of the environments where they were taught. For example, doctors who have only seen babies born to anesthetized mothers have a different conception of what newborn muscle tone should be than practitioners attending un-medicated mothers (Simonds, Rothman, and Norman 2006). What the traditional midwives at the Saber Nacer conference were demonstrating, then, were the ways that their knowledge about birth is shaped by the social, political, economic, and historical structures that inevitably affect women's bodies and health. When towns are too far from emergency hospital support, having a breech birth can mean serious complications or even death; in these towns, then, routine uterine massage intended to keep babies head down is an appropriate intervention that stems from local necessity and experience.

It makes sense that many of the elements of traditional midwifery made their way into the realm of more formalized, professional midwifery education; they were practices and treatments that had proven useful and that many patients expected from their midwives. But as these practices and treatments came into places like CASA and Mujeres Aliadas professional midwifery schools, they had to find their place alongside biomedical and other, globally derived alternative approaches. The result, I argue, was that traditional midwifery took on a new life guided by practitioner experience, patient desires, and necessity. The following account of a long prenatal consult I observed in the CASA midwifery clinic shows how these various care practices can intersect.

A Continuum of Care: Traditional Practices in Professional Midwifery

"This baby has *ni pies ni cabeza*" (neither feet nor a head), exclaimed Alejandra, a professional midwife working and teaching at CASA, as her hands gently palpated her patient's expansively pregnant belly. She then turned to glance over her shoulder, remembering that she had two first-year midwifery students observing her. Seeing their confused expressions, she held up her hands in a pose of surrender and quickly added, "Joke! Joke! You wouldn't really believe that it didn't have feet or a head, right?" The students gave forced chuckles, and Alejandra turned back to her patient. She explained that she could not feel the baby's position clearly because the uterus kept contracting into a hard ball (in a series of pre-labor contractions), making it difficult for her to feel anything. She suggested that they head over to the ultrasound room to get a clearer picture of the position, seeing as the woman was due any day and she wanted to know if the head was in the optimal position for labor.

We all marched down the hall to the ultrasound room; along the way, Alejandra quizzed the students on signs of impending labor. When we got to the small exam room, the technician squirted some gel from a repurposed yellow plastic mustard container onto the patient's abdomen, and we watched as the baby came into view on the small black-and-white screen. It quickly became clear that the baby was sideways rather than upside down. Its neck also arched strangely backward, which made the students laugh a little as they tried to contort their own necks to mimic this odd position. "Your baby is doing fine, except for this strange position. And it's a girl!" the technician told the patient with a grin. At this the patient pushed herself up to peer closer at the smudgy image on the screen, saying, "What? My doctor told me it is a boy!" to which the technician backtracked quickly, mumbling something about how she might be wrong, that she may have mistaken the anus for the vagina. The woman looked a bit unsettled by this confusing information, but Alejandra jumped in to discuss the issue of the position.

"We have to try to get this baby head down before you go into labor," she said. "Do you think your mother knows anyone in your *rancho* (rural community) that can do a sobada?" Alejandra asked. The patient shook her head, and Alejandra began to lament that the only traditional midwife on staff at CASA was home sick that day, when a student suggested that they ask Julieta, another staff midwife (whose story is discussed in Chapter 3 and in Dixon, El Kotni, and Miranda 2019). Julieta was not a traditional midwife; indeed, she was one of CASA's first graduating professional midwives and was back working at the clinic and teaching the students. However, the students had heard that she knew about sobadas—she had learned them from her mother when she was younger—and so we all made our way to Julieta's consult room. Julieta, a thirty-four-year-old woman with long hair and a grin that took up half her face, greeted us and listened as Alejandra described the situation; she would be happy, she said, to do a sobada. The patient smiled at her, reassured, and Julieta searched the room for an acceptable place to conduct the procedure.

During Alejandra's initial assessment of the patient during this consult, her inability to feel the baby's position with her hands led her to suggest the ultrasound. During the many consults I observed at CASA, conducting an ultrasound on a patient just to determine the position was rare; indeed, the midwives were usually quite confident about their ability to feel the baby with their hands. They would grasp the baby's head and gently wiggle it, noting whether it was engaged in the pelvis yet (a sign that labor may be immanent). Alejandra's decision to use the ultrasound was not based on an inability to feel for baby positioning in utero, but because the contractions were making the woman's uterus tight, and Alejandra did not want to hurt her by pushing around in there. The ultrasound was, then, a backup plan— not a necessary first step—used in this case to ensure the patient's comfort. The students, who followed Alejandra throughout this process, noted such informal protocols; when it came time for them to see their own patients, these experiences would influence their own decisions about when to use ultrasound technology.

Once the ultrasound technician brought the baby onto the screen—and confirmed its transverse alignment in the uterus—the students witnessed the conflicting potentials of the technology. On the one hand, the ultrasound was able to quickly illustrate the transverse position of the baby—a helpful tool that was being used as part of Alejandra's assessment of the patient. On the other hand, the biomedical authority attached to the machine and its technician was put into question when the technician misread the baby's sex. For the students, this slippage in the authority of a complicated and hard to understand technology was one example of the ways biomedicine becomes seen as a last resort. Students learned that biomedical, technological knowledge is not infallible, and they came to the consensus that it cannot be depended on alone. Alejandra's failure to ascertain the baby's position resulted from her desire to not hurt the patient; the failure of the ultrasound technician resulted from the technology and her reading of it.

Such moments remind us that biomedical technologies are not infallible and impersonal; rather, their use and interpretation depend on the people and institutions that have access to them. As Margaret Lock and Vinh-Kim Nguyen argue, we must pay attention to the ways that "the promise of and the actual effects of biomedical technologies are embedded in the social relations and moral landscapes in which they are applied" (2010, 5). As these student midwives go into the world as practitioners, their understanding and use of biomedical technologies could have significant impacts on the kind of prenatal care women receive.

Back in Julieta's consult room we each found a space to stand. The softest thing in the room was a narrow pink cushion taken from a chiropractor's bench that wasn't being used. "This will have to do," Julieta said as she arranged it on the floor. Julieta gently helped her pregnant patient lie down on it, making sure that her hips and back were on the cushion and letting her legs relax onto the ground. The midwife lowered herself to one knee, her long braid swinging over one shoulder as she leaned toward the woman. One hand resting on the patient's belly, she looked up and asked the two students who were eagerly awaiting this—their first—sobada if they could fetch her some oil. "What kind of oil?" the students asked, to which Julieta replied casually that "anything will do—as long as it is not the kind that could induce contractions. So . . . not *sábila* (aloe) and not *menta* (mint). Better something like *manzanilla* (chamomile). Also, bring hot and cold compresses."

While they waited for the students to return, Julieta gave the patient a capful of homeopathic pills, which they call *chochos*, to dissolve under her tongue, telling her that they would also help the sobada to be more effective. She explained to the patient that the ultrasound had shown that her baby was transverse, instead of head down, and that with so little time until her due date they needed to get the baby positioned correctly. When the students returned with a selection of small dropper bottles full of oils, Julieta picked one and dripped it onto the woman's basketball-sized belly. I noticed that the skin was so taut that it was slightly bruised in some places. With gentle but confident movements, Julieta began her massage, starting with broad circular sweeps with her hands around the baby. "The oil makes it easier to massage her," she explained to the students, "and makes it so I don't hurt her skin." The students leaned in, hardly blinking. This was neither a technique taught in their regular classes nor one they would get many chances to observe during their clinical rotations; the art of the pre-natal sobada was being lost, they told me. It was a traditional midwifery skill, but their own time spent learning with traditional midwives was limited— getting to learn it in the CASA clinic with Julieta was a lucky opportunity.

Julieta asked next for her Pinard (a low-tech instrument used to listen to the baby's heart rate that takes years of practice to use correctly) to make sure that the massage was not distressing the baby. Alejandra glanced around and, not seeing the Pinard, handed her an electronic handheld Doppler, which made the heart rate audible to all of us from a tiny microphone. "The baby sounds fine," she said, and continued her massage more rigorously now; she alternated a rocking motion of the entire belly with a pushing, swirling motion of her hands around the baby, encouraging it to shift its position. This went on for many minutes, as the woman gradually relaxed and her belly began to visibly change in shape as the baby's position changed. It looked like a giant fish rolling in her belly, I thought to myself. The woman must have felt something as it rolled and stretched, as her eyes widened and she smiled up at Julieta.

When Julieta slowed her massage, a student returned with hot and cold compresses, which Julieta had the student press onto the woman's abdomen, the cold toward the top and the hot toward the pelvis, "to convince this little baby to keep its head down where it is nice and warm—and not to go up to where it is too cold!" explained Julieta. She rocked back onto her heels, stretching out her arms and fingers. Then she picked up the Doppler again to check the heart rate now that the baby had been turned.

This step was crucial, she later told me, because sometimes during these external rotations, the baby may get tangled in its umbilical cord or get otherwise distressed. I thought back to the sobada demonstration from the Saber Nacer conference, and how the midwife had explained why she did not need a Doppler; these conflicting ideas of the limits of what you can do and know with your hands alone mapped onto the very different educations and work environments of the traditional midwife at the conference and Julieta, trained and working at CASA. Guessing where the heart should now be located, Julieta pressed one end of the Doppler to the woman's skin, but we heard nothing but a low static. She moved it slowly up and down, side to side, and we all stared, unblinking, at the patient's belly. Suddenly, the urgent beating of the heartbeat blared out at us, and we breathed out and smiled at each other. "The heart rate is slightly increased," Julieta told the woman, "but that is to be expected. Your baby is now head down!"

Alejandra, who was by now kneeling on the ground next to Julieta, joked with the patient that she would now have to spend the rest of her pregnancy "holding your belly tightly so that the baby cannot turn back down." Julieta laughed, but then said, seriously, that the woman would "still need to keep taking the homeopathic medicine to make sure the baby stays down." Her coworker agreed, telling the patient that "homeopathic medicine is magic, really—it is the vital spirit!" The students all nodded their heads; homeopathic remedies were often discussed among students and with some teachers at CASA as somewhat "magical" in their mechanisms for healing anything from a headache to a transverse baby.[3]

Getting up carefully, the two midwives helped the woman to her feet and led her to the ultrasound room; they wanted to get concrete proof for the patient—beyond what Julieta felt with her hands and what we all saw as the belly bulged and shifted—that the baby was indeed head down. The students called out to their classmates to come and see this, the verified results of a sobada, and the ultrasound room was soon packed with young faces, eager to witness the outcome of this rarely seen intervention. The ultrasound technician gave a little cheer, prompting all in the room to sigh happily, as she displayed on her screen the baby's head in the perfect position. "I am going to buy you a chocolate bar!" Alejandra told Julieta, who stood by modestly but could not help grinning. "And I will buy you another one if that head stays down until birth!"

Julieta explained that her work was not yet done, however, and she led the (now much larger) group of student onlookers back to her consult room and repositioned the patient on the pink cushion. "Now we need to do a *manteada* to make sure the baby stays down." The *manteada* is a technique in which the midwife rocks the woman back and forth, suspended under her back by a sheet or a *rebozo* (shawl), in order to gently rock the baby downward and into the correct position. "We know that the head is down, but the neck is still too flexed; this movement will help straighten the neck out," explained Julieta. The students looked at each other in excitement—first a sobada and now a manteada! Two traditional midwifery techniques to witness in one consult. They jostled to get a space to watch as Julieta slipped a sheet under the woman's back and rocked her back and forth for a few minutes. She told the woman that when she went home, she should practice crawling on her hands and knees as often as she could, which would also help to keep the baby in the right position.

Shaking her head, Alejandra told Julieta that she "never learned to do sobadas or manteadas; it takes so much wisdom to know when to do it and when not to! The traditional midwives are the ones who know how to do these things." Julieta explained that her mother always told her that babies should be massaged into the correct position. "Ah, I see," said her coworker. "You have it in your blood, then. The thing is, I am a midwife out of love, not from ancestry!"

The dramatic unfolding of events during the sobada—discovering the transverse position, massaging the baby into place, revealing its position on the ultrasound, and performing the manteada—created the sensation of witnessing a performance. This sensation was heightened by the accumulation of students who came to see the process and by Alejandra's clear enthusiasm for and deference toward Julieta's abilities. With the "success" proven first by Julieta's assessment of the baby with her hands and second by the ultrasound image, the sobada took on a miraculous quality. Mei Zhan (2009) describes the potential for such moments of "miracles" in traditional medicine to affect authoritative structures. Efficacies from the margins create stories of miracles, which then re-inscribe the power of the traditional knowledge itself.

Yet the authority held here by Julieta, and by the traditional midwifery knowledge she displayed, must be understood within a particular time and place. As Brigitte Jordan suggests in her work on midwifery models, "for any particular domain several knowledge systems exist, some of which, by consensus, come to carry more weight than others, either because they explain the state of the world better for the purposes at hand (efficacy) or because they are associated with a stronger power base (structural superiority), and usually both" (1997, 56). Jordan alludes to the potential for communities where parallel knowledge systems may exist and be viewed as equals, where practitioners are able to seamlessly move between them depending on their needs. In the consult described here, Julieta and Alejandra draw from a range of knowledge systems—traditional Mexican midwifery (the use of the sobada and manteada), alternative treatments (essential oils and homeopathic pills), and biomedical technologies (the ultrasound and the electronic Doppler). Their decisions were based on what they thought best for the patient, what they knew how to do, and what they had access to. This combination of training, pragmatism, and access could explain what happens in most medical encounters—even the most biomedical. In settings where resources are scarce or where patients may feel more comfortable with one style of treatment over another, the ability to draw on multiple modalities of healing and to employ preventative measures makes sense. All this is to say that traditional midwifery is a flexible set of practices, technologies, treatments, and ideologies with roots outside biomedicine, and its continued use across Mexico reflects contemporary midwives' diverse educational opportunities, patient populations, and occupational settings.

Some midwifery schools in Mexico foreground traditional midwifery (broadly defined) because of this diversity. Rather than viewing this as a situation in which, as Vega says, "humanized-birth techniques originating in the Global North are combined with 'traditional' methods through a New Age logic that confounds Euro-American notions of chronology and progress" (2018, 152), I argue that the schools' efforts to bring together various alternatives alongside biomedicine in the teaching of midwifery reflect an understanding that flexibility is necessary to the job.

This is the case at the Oaxaca City-based program to which I refer in this book as "Nueve Lunas," though its name has changed since my research to Centro de Iniciación a la Partería en la Tradición de Nueve Lunas (Center of Initiation to Midwifery in the Tradition of Nine Moons). The school expanded its name to more clearly indicate its relationship to traditional approaches; however, they did so in a way that signaled a more nuanced understanding of traditional midwifery. It is not a school that teaches students how to be traditional midwives; rather, it teaches them "midwifery in the tradition," which implies that the passing on of midwifery knowledge *is* the tradition, even if that knowledge may evolve over time. Indeed, that knowledge *must* evolve over time, to align with the needs of the modern patients being treated.

Teaching "Midwifery in the Tradition"

"Midwifery is supposed to be a varied, flexible profession; that is why it works," said Catrina, cofounder of Nueve Lunas. We were standing outside the classroom facilities while the students participated in a workshop with a traditional midwife named Carmelita, visiting from Cuernavaca. Together, we observed the students asking question after question, soaking in Carmelita's stories and teachings. The midwife was leading the students through a variety of topics, from general prenatal exam questions to problem solving in pregnancy. Some of her lessons were very hands on. At one point, for example, Carmelita demonstrated the use of *ventosas* (cupping) as a treatment for prenatal back pain. Students gathered round, taking notes and photos as she wiped some rubbing alcohol along the rim of a small glass, lit it on fire, then quickly set it on a student volunteer's back, extinguishing the fire and bringing blood to the area. One student asked her, "Isn't this originally a form of Chinese medicine?" Carmelita replied with a laugh, "I don't think my mother or my grandmother knew any Chinese people!" Indeed, the literature supports Carmelita's assertion that cupping has a long history in the Americas; however, like most therapies, it has traveled and meant different things to different people along the way (Elsubai and Aboushanab 2017). Later that day, the visiting midwife and teacher, Alison, would teach students how to analyze lab tests for their patients and make treatment decisions based on things like indications of infection. In these ways, students were receiving an array of types of training, filling their toolboxes with the diverse kinds of knowledge and skills they would someday need.

Back outside, the sun was hot on our shoulders, the adobe walls of the classroom warm against the bright blue sky. Catrina and her business partner, Amanda, began telling me about how they thought the future of midwifery education should look for Mexico. Amanda was from Mexico City and had become a midwife after training with Catrina, herself trained as a nurse midwife in her native Italy. Both were highly educated, experienced, and passionate about midwifery; like CASA's founder, Nadine, they were able to harness international interest because of their own cosmopolitan histories, yet they were also both quick to identify themselves as allies of local women. I had met them both years before, when we all got together to study women's health in small, borrowed spaces in downtown Oaxaca City, back before I went to graduate school and before they opened Nueve Lunas, back when we were all trying to figure out how to think about midwifery in Mexico. "Someone told me once that the very problem with midwifery in Mexico today is that it is not a well-defined field," Catrina said. "But I say . . . that is exactly where our strength lies." Her words were emphatic, but her tone was tired.

Amanda looked at me for a moment before asking, carefully, "You have been working with other midwifery schools. Do *you* think that the more professional midwifery education model will become the only model for Mexico?" I understood that this was a loaded question; on the one hand, it was a test of my trust and comprehension of the complexities of these competing visions for midwifery education, while on the other hand they really wanted to know what I perceived from my time with different organizations. "I don't know," I answered honestly. "I don't think it makes sense to view this as a competition between models of schools."

But for Catrina and Amanda, there *did* seem to be a race to determine which education model would win out in Mexico (the professional models like CASA or Mujeres Aliadas or the traditional models like Nueve Lunas), a dichotomous relationship that they also expressed in terms of what they called the homogenization of midwifery versus variability—or standardization versus multiplicity. For them, the idea of a standardized education program aligned with the state health-care system went against the tenants of midwifery itself. The first goal of their school was to facilitate the training of women who would carry on the local traditions and practices of midwives in their own villages. This necessarily implied, then, that even within the school, students would be learning different things depending on the knowledge of the midwives with whom they apprenticed. They came together for one week a month to do workshops and share experiences in Oaxaca City, but the rest of the time they were on their own, apprenticing with community-based, traditional midwives. The second goal was to preserve the knowledge and practices of traditional midwives. This was emphasized both through the structure of the apprenticeship model as well as through the teachings provided by visiting traditional midwives who came to the weekly classes to share their knowledge. These teachings were balanced by shorter biomedical trainings that introduced students to tools and concepts they might need to know in order to be flexible practitioners (such as how to read a lab test and how to take vital signs).

For Catrina and Amanda, the kind of midwifery education model that Mexico needed was one that allowed its graduates to be the most flexible.

This flexibility would entail the ability not only to practice according to the customs and needs of their individual communities but also to draw on accumulated internationally sanctioned knowledge and practices; in this vision, the two founders mirrored their own backgrounds as internationally savvy but locally focused practitioners. This model thus had students learn primarily from traditional midwives who already had community knowledge; the Nueve Lunas program served as a way to add to that knowledge and also create networks between students. In addition, Catrina noted that it made sense for the students to be accountable to a basic set of skills that all midwives should know, and that Nueve Lunas could help them learn these skills. But her concern was that, as CASA made strides with government recognition of professional midwives through official channels, less institutionalized forms of learning would soon become unacceptable to the state. "I worry that if CASA begins to open new schools across Mexico, they will become the only legal form of midwifery education in Mexico," Catrina told me. "For now, midwives still occupy a space outside of legality, for the most part. But any time one group gets defined as the legal form, others eventually become illegal by default."

Aside from questions about legality and regulation, Catrina argued that models like CASA just don't work for Mexico and its maternal health-care needs. "At CASA, they take students out of their home communities for three years! Studies have shown that if you do that, they won't go back to their communities," she argued. She went on to assert, as if quoting from such studies, that "only one in ten will return to her community," explaining that "three years away makes them too distant from their community, which is why we structured *this* program the way that we did." At Nueve Lunas, the students only come to the city for one week a month, and thus they maintain constant ties back home. Amanda jumped in to say that "midwives have always been leaders in their communities, so we want to maintain and support that idea."

"Come," said Catrina, "let's sit down." We climbed the steps back up to the doorway to the classroom, and Amanda went inside to get some work done. Inside, the students were practicing techniques that the visiting midwife had taught them, using rebozos to shift a baby's position in utero. They took turns playing the pregnant woman, laughing as they got on their hands and knees to let their partner wrap the rebozo under their belly and gently rock it back and forth.

We sat on the top steps, looking back over our shoulders at the students for a few moments. They came from all over—not only from the rural villages but also from nearby cities or even international locations. They all shared enthusiasm for what they were learning, and sounds of laughter and excitement could be heard from across the long classroom as they took turns pretending to be the pregnant woman and the midwife. We turned eventually, sitting beside each other but staring out toward the green mountains that surrounded the valley. Catrina looked tired to me, and worried, when we talked about the future of midwifery in Mexico.

The class inside got louder as the students broke for lunch, and we stood up to join them. "This is really hard," I said to Catrina, looking at the students but referring to her larger project of inserting the goals of Nueve Lunas into the goals of midwifery training nationwide. She understood me and sighed. "Yes," she said, "it is. But we cannot just focus on the idea that we have to solve it all today. We have to focus on the bigger picture." For Catrina and Nueve Lunas, this bigger picture was that midwifery should remain a profession of multiple possibilities for entrance and for practice, with as many kinds of midwives as there were kinds of women to become them. For them, this approach to midwifery education was the only one that made sense, the only one that was appropriate for Mexico. It emphasized the value of women's knowledge, of local knowledge, and the heterogeneity of women's needs across Mexico. It eschewed the idea that ties to the health-care system and formal state recognition were necessary to effectively train students.

Yet the students had other ideas about what would be appropriate for themselves as practitioners—and these ideas mostly had to do with their desire for some kind of certification, which would allow them to find jobs, get paid well, and be respected. Nueve Lunas did give graduates a *título*, which basically showed that they completed the curriculum, community service, and their thesis project. Catrina and Amanda told me that the título was not the point of the program but that all the students wanted one. "All of the graduates have it blown up and framed over their desks very proudly," they told me. Later, at a visit to one of the graduate's homes, I indeed noticed her framed título immediately upon entering. I asked her about it, and she laughed, saying that it was pretty but that it didn't mean anything, legally. What students wanted, more than this título, was the unattainable cédula profesional that CASA and Mujeres Aliadas had secured for their graduates—a license which would both legitimize them as practitioners and secure them employment. Catrina and Amanda understood why the students wanted this document, but they were conflicted about trying to get the school approved on that level. That was not what Nueve Lunas was meant to be about. They wanted the students' sense of authority to come from their knowledge and legitimacy in their communities, not from a state-granted piece of paper. Furthermore, even if they wanted to offer state certification, the route to getting cédulas for their graduates was complicated, unclear, and long. It also, noted Catrina, would require students to get a certain number of hours of clinical experience. "We have no desire to make our students get their clinical experiences in hospitals," Catrina said, scoffing at the idea. "Because, I mean, what are they going to learn there? Is *that* midwifery?"

For the founders of Nueve Lunas, midwifery was necessarily multiple in its definitions, yet these multiplicities had limits. That is, as Catrina implied, midwifery was *not* to be found in hospitals. The way Catrina thought schools should teach midwifery in Mexico, then, was to maintain the distinction between it and the biomedical practices that resided in hospitals. To maintain midwifery as a practice that was linked to communities, homes, women, and women's knowledge—in all these ways, she saw the elements of traditional midwifery as central to what midwifery is and does. Her vision necessitated a foundational respect for the knowledge and practices of traditional midwives, who all of my informants agreed were quickly dying out nationwide. An appropriate response to this phenomenon, according to Catrina and Amanda, then, was to train women who had intimate ties to these midwives in a way that ensured their ability to continue the legacies of flexible, community-based midwifery care.

Conclusion

Traditional midwifery in Mexico has changed and continues to change. Midwives who identify as traditional or employ traditional techniques must adapt to the changing needs of their patients and to the changing conditions in which they work. Even for those who view traditional midwifery as something that should exist outside the formal health-care system, complete separation from bureaucracy proves impossible. For, despite all the other services midwives offer, they do deal in life and death—topics that the state wants to control. The government has targets to hit and global agencies it is responsible to. Traditional midwives sometimes fit into the state's vision for how to achieve those targets, and sometimes they do not. The midwives I worked with had seen the pendulum swing enough times to realize that they would have to advocate for their own careers and find ways to work around barriers when the tide turned against them.

As schools like Nueve Lunas and individual midwives like Carmelita and Julieta continue to teach and employ traditional midwifery methods— broadly defined—they do so while pushing back against anti-traditional midwifery state policies or rhetoric. In many places, traditional midwives struggle to get birth certificates for their clients, causing them to have to create elaborate work-arounds (such as clients going alone to the government offices weeks later and claiming that they gave birth, unassisted, at home). Traditional midwives see the irony in the state's removal of their right to grant birth certificates while simultaneously holding them up as showpieces of Mexico's traditional roots when it serves the state's image. As one midwifery school administrator told me, "*Solamente las quieren para sus fotos*" (They only want them for their photos), referring to the ways that traditional midwives are often asked to dress up in their Indigenous outfits for promotional pamphlets.

Traditional midwives have long been seen by the Mexican medical field and the state alike as remnants of Mexico's romanticized history—remnants that reflect a precolonial past (and thus are interesting to showcase) but that also reveal the uneven reach of modernization through biomedical expansion. I describe in Chapter 1 how, since the 1850s, doctors in Mexico have been trying to curtail traditional midwives' practices, to discipline them into recognizing that they are "nothing more than special nurses" who should not be overextending themselves or taking on jobs that belong to doctors (Flores 1886, 576; my translation). Yet as traditional midwives still feel called to their work and responsible for their communities, they continue to find ways to practice.

I spent some of my time completing the writing of this book in Mexico, where I had a chance to catch up with many of the midwives discussed throughout these chapters. One lamented to me that in some parts of Mexico, traditional midwives are being offered money to basically serve as *anfitrionas* (hostesses) outside public hospitals to encourage their community members to come in. I was reminded of Nadine, from CASA, telling me about how midwives were once used as hooks to get women into hospitals and to trust biomedical practitioners. "Why are the midwives willing to do that?"

I asked my friend. She laughed, sadly, and said, "The traditional midwives are happy to be getting paid anything at all and to be recognized for their status in the community. The fact that they aren't being allowed to do any actual midwifery in those hospitals is secondary to that." Again, the midwives are being pragmatic, not dogmatic—they recognize the opportunity to work and be seen, even if it means not doing what they were trained to do.

This new manifestation of midwives' role as a bait to lure women into clinics and hospitals under the guise of interculturality is not unique: traditional midwives and other healing practices have been incorporated through many policies across Mexico in the name of tailoring health care to diverse cultures (Tucker et al. 2013). Lucia Guerra-Reyes (2019) notes that this trend extends across Latin America but describes how, in Peru, the new Intercultural Birthing Policy (which seemed to be a response to the desires of Indigenous women with whom Guerra-Reyes had long worked) has ultimately reproduced entrenched power dynamics between the state and Indigenous people and pushed women away from traditional home births. However, as in the case of Mexico, Guerra-Reyes recognizes Peruvian midwives' ability to "cannily" navigate shifting state priorities in order to continue to do their jobs (she also finds that some families do find ways to have the birth they want, despite official efforts that may stand in their way).

As global health agencies collect data, evaluate, and reexamine what roles traditional practitioners should play in health care, and as these determinations trickle down to local practitioners in cities like Oaxaca City, Pátzcuaro, San Cristobal de las Casas, or San Miguel de Allende, midwives continue to do what they need to do—for themselves and their communities. Even as the roles and identities of the traditional midwife will certainly continue to change in Mexico, the set of practices, technologies, treatments, and ideologies associated with traditional midwifery will most likely carry on because they are political, pragmatic, and modern.

Creating Demand and Demanding Change

Midwifery is changing in Mexico, as around the world; but then again, it has always been a dynamic profession. Through the process of researching and writing this book, I have seen the global community shift its stance on midwives and the Mexican government undergo various changes of heart when it comes to levels of official investment in midwifery training. Yet, as I have shown throughout these chapters, midwifery persists because it resists—while it simultaneously works alongside—the structures and systems that prevent women from getting the best quality of care. In short, midwives remain relevant because women still need them.[1]

In the Introduction, I asked why midwifery has not disappeared completely in places like Mexico, with its decades-long efforts to bring women into hospitals and to marginalize midwives. Through the chapters that followed, however, I ended up answering a slightly different question: rather than explain merely why midwives still exist in Mexico, I illustrated the reasons why they remain relevant. That is, I argue that midwifery persists because midwives occupy an important position in the health-services continuum: they are both insiders and outsiders, and they hold the potential to bridge the gap between the communities they serve and the health services these communities need. More importantly, they hold the potential to change the way women and women's health are viewed within the healthcare system and in society at large. They have to work both with and against the system as they strive to improve the quality of care while remaining accountable to the global community and its driving interests in measurable improvements in health outcomes.

This middle position that they occupy is not new. As described in Chapter 1, Mexican midwives have a long and complicated history of entanglements with the state. Further, their scope of practice and educational opportunities have long been affected by globally informed policies and ideologies. During colonialism, midwives across Spain's colonies were told that they had to become certified; the requirements of certification were set by far-away Spain—a fact that rendered them inappropriate for the contexts in which midwives were working. Years later, as midwifery education became a formal state project in independent Mexico, requirements such as French language skills revealed a continued disconnect between what midwives did and were and what the state wanted them to do and be.

Yet as I have argued here, rather than simply becoming fully absorbed into the state health-care system or fully disappearing from the medical landscape, midwives have used this middle ground to get their work done. They have continued to advocate from a platform of social justice for systemic and infrastructural changes to support better health access and quality of care, while simultaneously addressing national and global health priorities through their labor and advocacy. In Chapter 2, I showed how maternal mortality reduction has become a central focus of global health initiatives and, consequently, a central interest of the Mexican government. By tracing the ways that Mexican midwives have embraced this pressing concern while strategically linking their own goals for improving the quality and breadth of care in women's health, I highlighted the utility of existing in such a middle space.

Because of their insider/outsider status, midwives have a unique position from which to critique the way biomedical health care is delivered in Mexico and beyond. In Chapters 3 and 4, I discussed the issues of infrastructural and obstetric violence and showed how they both arise out of larger contexts of social inequality and, particularly at this time, national insecurity. As midwives address the conditions women face that may set them up to receive poor health care or suffer poor health outcomes, they firmly plant midwifery as a social justice intervention as well as a medical one. Midwifery, they argue, offers both a viable educational and career option that can give back to communities and a level of health-care provision that is flexible, able to address the needs of marginalized communities, and cost effective. Midwives can go where doctors cannot or will not go; they can bridge the gap between rural villages and faraway health-care centers. Midwifery is an important part of the puzzle of health-care delivery. Perhaps most importantly, they argue, they can offer a more humane form of treatment that can qualitatively improve women's experiences with care—which may also lead to measurable improvements in health outcomes. By offering respectful women's health care, midwives hope to improve women's trust in providers, increase the attention women get to their health and well-being across their lifespan (not only in the moment of childbirth), and empower them to make choices about how they want their birth to proceed. Such changes are inherently tied to a social justice agenda, in that they address the root causes of health disparities and propose a leveling solution that gives all women agency and access to care.

While the bulk of my research was conducted with midwives who were training or working at established midwifery schools across Mexico, I did not want to leave the voices of traditional midwives out of this book. First, this was because of how entangled the ideas of traditional midwifery practices were in all forms of midwifery. Whether they were called "professional" or "traditional," the kinds of midwifery I saw being practiced and taught inevitably gave recognition to and drew heavily on the practices and ideologies of traditional midwifery. In addition, I came to understand that, rather than (only) referencing Mexico's Indigenous past, traditional midwifery is also a very dynamic, modern concept; it uses the tools available to treat modern bodies affected by modern health issues and constrained by modern structures and society.

The International Day of the Midwife

Even as I have tried here to tease apart all of the ways that midwifery matters in Mexico, I recognize that such arguments need to be fully embraced by the people midwives hope to serve as well as the governments who hold the power to shape midwifery's future. This has been an uphill battle in many ways for the midwives I worked with. Midwifery is seen by some as, at best, old fashioned—or, at worst, dangerous. Others simply do not know what midwives can do. Given the changing formats of midwifery education in Mexico, it is understandable that most people may not know what it means for a midwife to have gone to a formal education program or what differences among types of licensure could signify. As the midwives I worked with settle into their careers, open new schools, continue to organize with each other, and bring attention to the work that they do and the efforts they fight for, they need to generate buy-in from their communities and their government.

However, changing how people think about birth in Mexico and beyond is going to take some doing. Not only would local, state, national, and global policy makers need to clarify routes for midwifery training and protect their scope of practice, but women and families would also need to view mid-wives as a viable option for health care. Midwives would need to become seen as desirable both because of their ability to safely manage low-risk births and because of their humanistic approach to their patients. But how could such changes come about, especially given the decades of emphasis on hospital births and marginalization of midwifery?

This question weighed heavily on all of the midwifery schools where I spent time during my research. They were struggling to get funding, institutional backing, and at least some level of recognition for the good work they were doing. But perhaps most of all, they were trying to reach the populations they aim to serve, to educate them on their options, and to convince them to see the benefits of midwifery. As I observed during classroom conversations; administrative meetings with local, state, and federal officials; activist conferences; and patient consults, I watched this work unfold—the slow and multi-pronged attempts to build support for midwives. One day, late in my fieldwork in 2012, captured many of the facets of this work.

It was the International Day of the Midwife, and CASA's midwifery school had gone all out in celebration. The school—itself a lovely set of buildings with arched porticos and courtyard gardens—sat atop a hill overlooking the picturesque city of San Miguel de Allende. That day, busloads of people from nearby communities had been brought in for the celebration and sat expectantly in rows of folding chairs in CASA's main hall—a grand, two-story space that had been festooned with ribbons and balloons. Tables with *jamaica* water and small paper cups of sliced jicama and carrots with lime, salt, and chili were set out for attendees. Television and radio crews set up around the periphery, alerted by the school that state officials would be there. While they waited for the politicians, they interviewed CASA mid-wives and took photographs. Children ran around playing in the gardens outside. Some CASA students sat in neatly pressed school uniforms along the back wall, while the rest of the students left to set up an outpost at the city park down the hill.

The meeting was opened by CASA's director, who gave moving remarks about the need for midwifery today. With tears in her eyes, she scanned the crowd and implored them to consider midwifery as a beautiful and caring profession but also as an important one. "It is a *shame* that women keep dying in their births in Mexico. A shame," she repeated, heavily. "But international studies show that midwives can reduce this maternal mor-tality—so here we are!" She ended her opening on a high note but with a clear message: maternal health is suffering, and midwifery can be part of the solution.

The speakers that followed the director had been driven into town that morning, and their presence itself sent a strong message to the assembled crowd: midwifery was an issue important enough to bring state and national politicians to this small school to speak to the people. First to speak was Dr. Susana Cerón, the general director of the National Center for Gender Equity and Reproductive Health. She quickly and succinctly gave modern midwifery some historical context: she explained how the shift in the mid-twentieth century of birthing in hospitals improved health outcomes for some, but many communities still suffered high rates of maternal mortality. "In countries like ours," she said, looking out over the crowd, who perhaps knew this already but who also perhaps appreciated hearing her say it, "there are very dramatic contrasts. Some communities are very far from health services in Mexico, especially rural and Indigenous communities, and this can lead to more problems in birth." Cerón went on to talk about how the World Health Organization supported trained birth attendants like midwives as a way to bring care to marginalized communities by addressing low-risk pregnancy and birth. "But we need more. And that is why CASA and schools like it are so important." At this, everyone cheered. Cerón looked out at everyone, and when they quieted down, she said, in a more thoughtful tone:

> The secretary of health in Mexico cares about reducing maternal mortality. But something we don't think about a lot is the notion of humanized birth. That is, we don't talk much about the benefits of women having a natural birth, of reducing cesarean rates—which is a huge abuse of the health services—promoting lactation, or strengthening family bonds. Yes, we want to train providers who have the technical knowledge to work in hospitals, but we also need this humanized aspect of care. That is why we are so proud of CASA at the secretary of health office. I think that this model here could be reproduced all over the country. And I think that it is especially necessary to strengthen and reproduce this model in this time, while we are committed to reducing maternal mortality.

Cerón's speech was short but significant in its layers. She established her authority as a national government representative, summarized the legacies of inequality in Mexico that have led to unequal health outcomes, clearly linked midwifery education to maternal mortality reduction, and made the case for the humanization of care. As such, her brief speech had broad appeal.

Next to speak was perhaps the most anticipated guest, Secretary of Health for the State of Guanajuato, Dr. Juan Luis Mosqueda. Just prior to the formal presentation, I had listened as he and CASA founder Nadine had hashed out some of Nadine's complaints about the state's support for midwifery, and I had seen Mosqueda take in her concerns with a mixture of agreement and bemusement. Nadine was frustrated that the state sometimes gave lip service to the idea of supporting midwives while denying them the ability to have a reasonable scope of practice—for example, limiting the types of contraception they could offer. Nadine's list of demands for Mosqueda was long, and while he tried to appease her in their meeting, I could not tell whether he actually meant what he said. It was with some surprise, then, that I listened to Mosqueda extol the virtues of midwifery to the assembled audience during his presentation. In contrast to his slightly defensive, deer-in-the-headlights attitude during the previous meeting, Mosqueda described the state's support for midwifery in clear and moving terms. He said:

> It is great to be here on the International Day of the Midwife. There is nothing more beautiful than the beginning of life—and nothing more gratifying than the people who accompany our women when they give birth. It is very worrisome that we have maternal mortality rates so high . . . unfortunately, we will never be able to get them down to zero. But they are still higher than we want them to be. We must understand that maternal mortality must be addressed from different angles. . . . Maternal mortality could be reduced if we worked with women from the beginning. Here, all of this is relevant: Communities work on this, institutions like CASA work on this, midwives work on this . . . and this work, it goes beyond just technical knowledge—the knowledge of skills they can do—it is also the emotional accompaniment in pregnancy and birth that matters and also all the work of sensitization and education about the next pregnancy, family planning, and lactation. All of this together is really what favors the reduction of maternal and infant mortality. Like Cerón said, I feel very proud to have CASA here in the state. Because it really is an area we need to work on. And we have to work together. CASA works to assure that the people who train as midwives have the right knowledge—but they also need to know that they have our backing. If you [midwives] need support for an emergency, you can count on us and know that the communication lines are open. We all have the same goal—reduce maternal mortality.

Like Cerón, Mosqueda framed the state's support of midwifery in rela-
tion to maternal mortality reduction, while recognizing briefly the other
"emotional" work that midwives can do. As I have discussed throughout
this book, these two emphases—to reduce maternal deaths and humanize
care—play important roles in the dissemination of midwifery in Mexico, as
elsewhere. Midwives and their advocates hear messages from politicians
like Cerón and Mosqueda and mirror them in their own advocacy. The
clear message being sent on that International Day of the Midwife was that
maternal mortality was the primary national concern; humanization of care
was secondary, if, as they recognized, connected. Nadine's frustration in
her earlier meeting with Mosqueda came out of the frustrations midwives
nationwide had expressed: to them, humanized care was the basis for better outcomes, including reduction in maternal deaths. Instead of an afterthought, it had to be the basis for systemic change.

The two arguments that I have woven through this book are, first, that
the conditions for care in Mexico condition women to accept and experience poor treatment and bad outcomes and, second, that midwives are con-
sciously trying to work both with and against state, national, and global
health policies in an effort to change those conditions. As global priorities
for women's reproductive health care shift and become codified in changing
initiatives, goals, and publications, their impacts trickle down to national
and state levels. Midwives in Mexico have seen enough of these changes to
recognize that they need to be flexible and savvy to the fickle interests of the
government while also building a base of support that can withstand such
changes. They need to make their relevance clear and change the underlying structures by building themselves into them.

Cerón's and Mosqueda's show of support reflects the slow entrance of
midwifery into state and national policy, though midwives argue that there
is much more work to be done if midwifery is to be protected and made
available to all women. On the state level, Veracruz and Guerrero have thus
far incorporated midwifery into their policies on maternal health, while a
handful of federal agencies have also shown some level of interest in, at
the least, professional midwifery. However, despite national representatives
like Cerón presenting a clear show of support for midwifery in Mexico, the
federal government has not been consistent in its advocacy for midwives of
any sort. Thus, even as "states are successfully advancing midwifery models
of care without a national-level mandate, state-level officials claim the lack
of a mandate makes the road more difficult and leaves the sustainability of

their programs in question" (Atkin et al. 2019, 29). One potential reason for this lag in government support is the continuing lack of consensus among midwifery groups (such as those described in this book) about how certification should work, what role perinatal or obstetric nurses should play, and the appropriate levels of training and scopes of practice of professional and traditional midwives (Atkin et al. 2019).

And so this tension continues, between the desire on the part of some for midwifery to remain a-legal, autonomous, and self-sufficient and the push by others to institutionalize midwifery in some fashion so that it is sustainable, regulated, and accessible. This controversy stems in part from a question I heard debated by various individuals to different ends: can midwifery retain its flexible, humanized approach to women and communities if the state mediates what "counts" as midwifery knowledge and regulates what midwives can and cannot do? On the one hand, some midwives point to the state's current interest in adding midwifery to nursing schools as a sign that midwifery itself is being grossly underappreciated and coopted, turned into something it is not. On the other hand, some argue that the only way for midwifery to survive an expanding health-care system and become an option for more women is to work with the state, even if that means that, in the process, its essence may change over time. Lisa Mills (2010) has argued that the kinds of reproductive rights that countries like Mexico signed on to champion at the Cairo conference in 1994 can be the real rights of a nation's citizens only when the state actively takes them on to safeguard. It remains to be seen whether and how the Mexican government will safeguard maternal health by investing in midwifery on a larger scale.

While midwives and midwifery schools were doing the work of meeting with politicians, justifying their existence through their ability to reduce maternal mortality and improve health outcomes, and securing legitimacy through government licensure, they took a different strategy in trying to shift the perspective of the communities they served. As Cerón noted, and as the midwives were well aware, women had been urged for half a century to deliver their babies in hospitals under the promise of better outcomes. Trying to convince people to reconsider midwives as a safe and humane alternative was hard work.

The International Day of the Midwife closed with a theater production, written by the CASA theater group in collaboration with the midwifery school, that illustrated very clearly the message midwives wanted Mexican families to receive: women should be allowed to choose where they want to

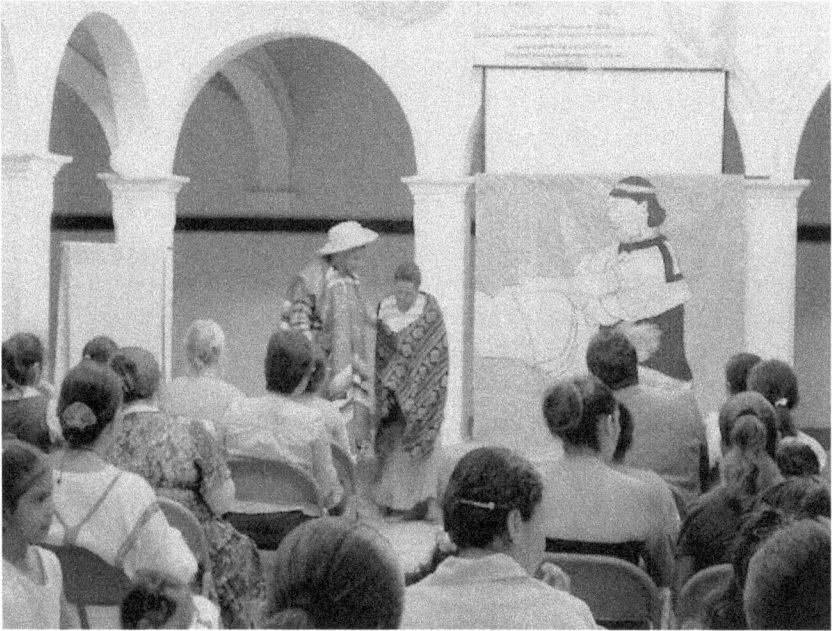

FIGURE 11: In this scene from *La vida en tus manos*, María and Pedro go in search of their local midwife. Photo by author.

receive their health care and deliver their babies, and making that choice based on a desire to feel respected is valid.

The play, titled *La vida en tus manos* (Life in your hands), was debuting at this event—an ideal location in which to start spreading its message, as the audience was a mixture of community members, politicians, and the media (see Figure 11). Later, the play would hit the road and be performed around the country, one effort among many to try to change how people thought about midwives and women's agency in choosing health-care providers (Jiménez 2012). The play and the narrative and counter-narrative it offered provided clear insight into the perspective of the CASA community and offered emotion-driven context for the audience to better understand why CASA's mission mattered. (This style of theatrical activism has been applied to various topics around the world; see, for example, Winskell et al. 2013 for an analysis of narrative performance on HIV in Southeastern Nigeria).

The podium was pushed to one side, and a makeshift theater was created by unfurling a painted banner depicting an Indigenous midwife and birthing women. A bed was rolled out carrying a sleeping couple, María and Pedro. They were dressed to appear as rural *campesinos* (farmers)—identities indicated by their worn leather sandals and simple cotton clothing and by María's shawl and Pedro's straw hat. As they slept, music started playing, and two actors danced out onto the stage—one held a large ovum, and the other held multiple sperm swinging around on long sticks. In tune with the music, the gametes danced around each other, until finally the ovum stuck to one of the sperm, and they danced off stage together as the music faded.

On the other side of the stage, the local midwife was kneeling and grinding corn on rocks with her daughter as she talked to her about becoming a midwife. Back in their bedroom, María emerged from the bed with a large belly, and she and Pedro hugged joyfully. She contacted the midwife to tell her about the pregnancy, and the midwife congratulated them.

Suddenly, a doctor and nurse showed up at the house and barged in. They began to speak rudely to the couple: they would need to have their baby with them at the hospital, because "as you see, now we have health for everyone," a nod to the idea that "health" is solely located in and distributed by the state. María said she was not sick, just pregnant, but the doctor laughed and said that was even more of a reason to go to the hospital. "But it is far. We don't have money," María replied. The doctor assured her the state would send people to check on her periodically and that it was important to get to the hospital for the birth so that her baby could get enrolled in the national health insurance program and be protected for life. This speech echoed the messaging that providers and workshops across Mexico dole out to women: hospitals are the only safe place to give birth (Miranda 2015). The couple was eventually convinced, and they told the midwife they had decided to go the hospital route. The midwife graciously bowed out, saying they should do what they felt was best.

Once María went into labor, the scene shifted to the hospital. She was given a paper face mask and told to lie down on a narrow bed. The nurse and doctor each briskly checked her cervical dilation as she writhed in pain. The doctor told her she still had a long way to go and sent her away. María said it hurt too much to go away at that point, so the doctor said to his nurse, "You know what? I think we should do a cesarean. These first-time moms fight too much, so surgery will be better." María tried to argue, and finally the doctor just said to go away and walk around, since they did not have any beds available, but to come back in three hours to see if there was an open bed by then. This was the turning point of the story. María had finally had enough; she was in pain and felt like the hospital that had promised a safer birth was falling short. She told her husband to take her back to their village and their midwife.[2]

The scene changed again as the couple approached the midwife, who welcomed them back and encouraged the husband to stay with his wife as she massaged María's belly and sang to them. The baby was born in an emotional moment—a doll emerged from under María's dress—and the couple thanked the midwife profusely. Pedro told her, "The truth is that I never thought about how each of us was born once and that we should all be born under good conditions, like our baby." María agreed, saying, "Women give life, and we have the right to have dignified treatment before, during, and after the birth . . . and *always*." The midwife chimed in with the sentiment that "a child who is born well will always be a good person." At this, the actors bowed to a standing ovation.

La vida did the work of highlighting both the potential of empowering women as the protagonists of their own births and the potential for midwifery to support this narrative shift. María begins the play with agency, choosing her local midwife to attend her birth. She is coerced into going to the clinic instead, where she quickly loses her power—a process documented through a series of stark visual and theatrical effects: her mouth is covered and muted with a surgical mask, and she is acted upon as the staff briskly check her cervical dilation. Her autonomy is further diminished as the doctor decides to do a cesarean without explaining himself to María or consulting her at all. In the space of a five-minute hospital scene, we see how quickly María disappears. It is the presence and promise of the village midwife that brings María's agency back into the story, as she makes the decision with her husband to leave the clinic and seek out a more respectful environment for her birth.

Further, the play explicitly makes the link between better birth experiences and better outcomes for women, children, and society. In naturalizing this link, the play adds urgency to the campaign to prioritize women's experiences and transforms the birth narrative from one that focuses solely on the mechanics of labor to one that situates birth within a broader social context. Theater can bring attention to the possibilities for power in intimate settings, as it allows the audience to engage publicly with issues thought of as private (Daniels 2015). In this way, it offers a parallel to the classic Mexican community productions of the *Posada* and *Pastorela*, ritualized retellings of the birth of Jesus in which we see how birth can sometimes unexpectedly change the world.

After the play was over, the celebrations continued down the hill in the town's central park, where a group of CASA's midwifery students were trying to reach out to the public and educate them about what midwives can do. A red tent had been erected and filled with cushions, rugs, and a small altar, where one of the midwives was doing *limpias* (spiritual cleansings) on anyone who was interested, using a dish of smoking fragrant copal (an aromatic tree resin used ceremonially). Some of the students were gathering pregnant women and giving them short informational talks and offering healthy foods and fruit water to passersby to entice them to stay and listen. They spoke about the CASA midwifery program but also more generally about why families might consider hiring a midwife for their reproductive health needs. They spoke of humane and respectful care, of allowing women to birth in the space where they felt comfortable and with the people they wanted to be near. They even spoke of the economic benefits of choosing a midwife (compared to paying a private doctor, a midwife was much cheaper). What they did not speak about to the assembled locals was the connection between midwifery and maternal mortality reduction.

I mention this because it stood in contrast to the formal presentation earlier in the day. To me, this distinction was one more example of the ways that midwives could switch gears between defending their profession in terms of its potential to address global health priorities and its potential to improve the quality of care for women.

As the student blew the copal smoke up and down women's bodies, she evoked ideas of traditional midwifery, even as she promoted herself as a professional midwife and spread the word to attendees about the professional midwifery school and clinic up the hill. The tent, the pillows, the rugs, the copal—these elements all caught people's attention. They seemed to say: be comforted here; here, you will be taken care of. Care will involve comfort and ritual and good food and support. These images represented the kinds of practices many students wanted to someday create, and they stood in stark contrast to the spaces and elements of public hospital rooms where most of the women walking by might have previously experienced labor. But would such imagery and outreach—or indeed, even formal government talks about the impacts of midwives on maternal mortality—shift the way people thought about midwifery?

Creating Demand for Midwifery

I was talking recently with CASA's founder, Nadine, about the ways that Mexican midwifery has changed over the last few decades and how midwives have carved a place for themselves in the health-care system by offering things that other providers cannot. I said, impassioned, "Midwifery matters now more than ever." She considered my words for a moment then asked me pointedly, "Matters to whom? To the government? To women? To men?" When I did not respond right away, she continued, "The government doesn't really care about midwifery per se; they don't really get it—they want maternal mortality to go down, but they don't fully understand what midwives do. Men don't want midwives; they don't want women to have choices with their reproductive health. And women—not even all women want midwives." When I asked her what she meant, she explained that in most parts of Mexico, women do not even know that they have the option of going to a midwife; they do not know that things could be different, that they could be treated better and have more choices in their care. She said that, while midwifery in Mexico has indeed gained visibility and legitimacy in many ways, it remains on the fringes of society. Upper-class women in cities may hire midwives because it is the trendy thing to do. Poor, marginalized women in rural communities go to midwives because there are no other options. Those few who have access to a professional midwife, trained at one of the schools described in this book, may fall somewhere in between. But what we need, Nadine argued, is for midwifery to be a viable option for all women. That is what CASA and the other schools were trying to do, albeit from small beginnings. To get to the kind of scale Nadine imagined, she said that women needed to be taught about what they were missing— you cannot demand what you do not even know is an option, she explained.

Nadine's words reminded me of a conversation I had with a CASA alumna, Alma, who had been doing workshops for pregnant women at a state-run medical clinic. Alma had told me about how hard it was to hear from women the ways that they believed they could get the best care during their labor and birth: the secret to a good birth, they told her, was to quietly endure, doing whatever the doctor or nurse tells you to do. Alma said that when she began telling these women about how they could be treated, about the choices and agency they could have in birth, they were originally skeptical. Then she showed them the national Mexican Norms that outlined explicitly the things that women are entitled to in labor—including the ability to have their partner with them, to birth in a vertical position if desired, and to expect protection against obstetric violence (Secretaría de Gobernación 2016). Alma said that when the women saw the official national expectations for how women should be treated in labor—and saw how different it was from their own experiences—"their eyes were opened." The women wrote comment cards demanding that the clinic adopt the national norms, and they planned to continue meeting and learning more about their rights.

While Alma's intervention was small and localized, it symbolizes the larger potential of midwifery in Mexico. Midwives can connect their communities to health services, but they can also educate women about their rights and promote a different model of care, in which women have choice and voice. This sentiment was summarized in a phrase I heard throughout my fieldwork: the argument that women need to become the "protagonists" of their own births (see Dixon 2020 for an in-depth analysis of this phrase). Midwives wanted to change the narrative about what mattered in health, how health care should be delivered, and the roles women and communities should play in their own health decision-making. In the counter-narrative they proposed, midwifery played an important role: midwives were writing themselves into the future they proposed for safer, more quality care.

If the effects of midwives and supporters' efforts are going to be felt by the vast majority of the population, however, the number of trained midwives will have to increase substantially. Indeed, as those who suffer the most from inhumane care and obstetric violence are often already from marginalized segments of the population, midwifery will need to become a viable option for those who enter into poor hospital conditions because they do not have another choice. A recent opinion piece in the *Washington Post* titled "Parir in México es un acto de resistencia" (Giving birth in Mexico is an act of resistance) points out that the conversation should not be about whether water births or home births are better or worse than hospital births but rather about giving women the ability to choose what they want for their own births. "Behind every midwife, doula . . . or mother who gives advice to another, there is a political position," writes journalist Alejandra Sánchez Inzunza (2020; my translation), whose own pregnancy and birth in Mexico provoked her to proactively try to avoid the horror stories she had heard from other women and read in the data by informing herself and advocating for what she wanted. Getting the word out that women even have options to investigate, and the opportunity to voice their concerns and desires to their providers, requires systemic change.

Midwifery is only one part of the solution to improving women's health care worldwide, but I argue it is an important part. As this book has described, not only are midwives able to offer humane, quality care to women and among communities, often in areas where there is little access to good care without them, but they also are able to stand up to the deeper injustices that lead to inequalities in health outcomes. This dual role is not limited to midwives in Mexico; indeed, Dána-Ain Davis found that while radical birth workers in the United States, including Black midwives and doulas, "may serve as a bridge in laboring and birthing processes, many believe that they should also participate in transforming the systems that place women and their children at risk" (2019, 197). Not all of the midwives I interviewed and spent time with desired a politically active life of critiquing the system or pushing back against inequities; many wanted to keep their heads down and deliver babies, tend to their clients, and live good lives. Yet collectively, the work they did was not carried out in isolation. From the tools and treatments used to the training received to the health issues they encountered, midwives were necessarily drawing on global webs of knowledge and practice while responding to the needs of modern bodies shaped by modern global politics. When midwives called for women to become the protagonists of their own births, their subtle but strong message was that we need to change the script.

In Chapter 1, I discussed the image of Mexican midwives being used historically as *ganchos* (hooks) to get women to go to hospitals for their care. Midwives were used in this way because of their ability to connect with patients and communities, to build trust, and to convince people that hospitals were safe and necessary. The hospitals needed the midwives to do this work, just as midwives have needed hospitals to give them places to practice, backing, and authority. Originally, the plan seemed to be to use midwives as hooks and then do away with them once hospitals became the norm, once midwifery became irrelevant. Yet decades later, midwives remain and continue to advocate for their own relevancy. They have dug in their heels and are using the goals and policies of global health to get themselves in the door, planting seeds of humane treatment and respect along the way.

"Peace on Earth Begins with Birth"

Ten years after meeting Juana and Elena (the midwives I discuss in the Introduction) at a national midwifery conference in Oaxaca, I found myself looking for them at another midwifery conference, this time in San Cristobal de las Casas, Chiapas (I discuss this conference in more detail in Chapter 5). I was there in my official ethnographer capacity, but I was also there as a peer of sorts this time—I knew many of the midwives who showed up (though I never did see Juana or Elena there), after a decade of working in women's health in Mexico. This meeting, held in 2010, felt like a pivotal moment for building the necessary momentum to bring midwives together from across the country and push for more recognition and legitimacy, as well as for organization among themselves.

Outside the main hall for the conference there was an area with tables set up for vendors to sell their wares; homemade salves in plastic tubs, homeopathic remedies in brown glass vials, dried herbal teas, woven *rebozos*, and baked goods were all stacked in lovely displays. Representatives from the different midwifery schools that I was studying were there, and I watched as women read through brochures, asked questions. I stopped by one of the booths, run by a midwife I knew from Oaxaca, and picked up a bright purple bumper sticker. *"La Paz en el Mundo Empieza con el Buen Nacer,"* it read. She saw me holding it and said, in English, the translation of the bumper sticker: "Peace on Earth Begins with Birth!"

I had heard the expression before, but it struck me at that moment that such a short and catchy, bumper-sticker-worthy rhyme might actually summarize the message the midwives were trying to convey. They are making the case that midwifery has the potential to do more than just help women have babies. A good birth, they argue, both reflects and reinforces a social dynamic in which women are valued and cared for, no matter what their background or skin color or class. Midwifery, argue the midwives, is more relevant than ever because midwives help improve women's births and women's lives more broadly. In a time of widespread social violence across Mexico, stubbornly high maternal mortality ratios, and widening divisions between the rich and the poor along racial and class lines, midwifery offers a corrective with the radical potential to change Mexico and, maybe, the world.

To be salable to government officials and policy makers in Mexico and beyond, this vision has to translate from the groovy bumper-sticker phrase to real, actionable ideas with lasting results. What would it mean—and what would it *take*, in a practical sense—for birth to be a transformative site? Scholars have argued that one way to address systemic inequality in health is to provide access to a range of reproductive health-care options, including midwifery, such that women can find the culturally *and* medically appropriate type and level of care for their needs (Goode 2014; Davis 2019). For Mexico, this means that "diversity—in the context of inequality—must be honored if midwifery is to be accepted in the regions that need it the most" (Atkin et al. 2019, 56). Alongside this diversity of options, collaboration is also necessary: to create real systemic change, midwives and the kinds of care they offer must be in some way connected to the health-care system: "The data show that the best maternal health outcomes are seen in places where midwives are integrated into teams of practice with clear and complementary roles" (Atkin et al. 2019, 56). Each school described in this book has tried to figure out what such integration should or could look like, while they have collectively been building a base of alternative care providers.

If birth is to be a site of real systemic change, then, birth workers like midwives cannot only work with or against the existing health-care system; they will have to continue to do both. They will need to continue to fight to change the ways women's health care is delivered and made available, while also building ever-stronger networks of support, sources for referrals, and systems of sustainability. While I was conducting this research, the tensions presented to me by midwifery students and school administrators were often framed in terms of a simple dichotomy: to work with the system or not. Yet for conditions to improve for all women, Mexico needs midwives to continue to do both. To keep one foot inside and one outside. To change the system from the inside while continuing to exert pressure from the outside, doing the exhausting work of ever pushing for better care.

NOTES

PROLOGUE

1. A doula is someone who supports a woman before, during, and after birth (DONA n.d.).
2. The honorific *Doña* is used to convey respect, often for an elder female; I have maintained the term *Doña* when others used it commonly to refer to that person. I have not used it when I did not hear others refer to a person using the term. Most names have been changed to pseudonyms throughout this book to protect their confidentiality, except for Nadine Goodman and Alison Bastien, who each asked to retain their names, and public officials.
3. See Dixon (2019) for a discussion of how my birth and early parenthood in Mexico came to impact my fieldwork.

INTRODUCTION

1. See (Dixon, Smith-Oka, and El Kotni 2019) for a more extensive discussion of the learning process among differently trained birth workers in Mexico.
2. Shakespeare wrote about *cardo santo*, which he called "Carduus Benedictus" and "plain holy-thistle," in *Much Ado about Nothing*. It was recommended by one character to another to heal the qualms of the heart (2005, 3.4.66-73).
3. While I recognize that the "state" has been conceptualized and defined in varying ways by anthropologists, I use the term in this book to generally refer to government entities, including local, state, and federal.
4. See Mills and Davis-Floyd (2009) for a detailed discussion of CASA's history.
5. Nadine Goodman requested that I use her real name in this text.
6. This goal of returning practitioners to rural regions from whence they came echoes efforts in the 1930s to train rural citizens in two-year rural medical programs and send them back to their communities; these efforts were highly critiqued as substandard at the time (Soto Laveaga 2013) but reflect the ongoing concern with training rural health providers who will remain in rural regions.
7. While CASA's graduates are officially "technical" midwives because of the name of their degree level, I refer to them here as "professional" midwives, which is how they primarily refer to themselves.
8. The state where CASA is located, Guanajuato, is still seen nationally as one of the most conservative states, and midwives would often refer to the state's "backward" nature, citing influences of the religious right within the state government on policies related to women's

health and reproduction. For example, CASA's consistent emphasis on family planning set off alarm bells for the predominantly conservative local officials, who raised issues with birth control and hinted at rumors of illegal abortions. Nadine complained bitterly during one meeting about how the state government was using state funds to distribute pamphlets in public schools disparaging the use of contraception. During my fieldwork, rumors of illegal abortions connected to CASA were blamed on malevolent government tactics to undermine the midwives' work, and multiple women were arrested and convicted for homicide when they went to the hospital during a miscarriage, a trend described elsewhere in Mexico (Mills 2010).

CHAPTER 1

1. Empirical midwives are generally defined as midwives who learn by experience or through apprenticeships (Mills and Davis-Floyd 2009), but they may also be seen in parts of Mexico as "mestiza women who are not legitimately recognized by the state as being registered or qualified" (Murray de López 2015, 5).

2. While Díaz was interested in science as a form of European modernity, the *científicos* (scientists) he was surrounded by were not necessarily actual scientists but rather positivists influenced by French intellectual Auguste Comte, who in turn influenced Díaz's thinking about ideas of social progress (Coerver, Pasztor, and Buffington 2004, 143).

3. This seems ironic in hindsight, as the physicians at that time were doing things in birth like bleeding the pregnant and postpartum women or using the "Playfair" method (which involved putting fingers into the woman's anus during labor to speed up birth) (Carrillo 1998).

4. This push to bring health and hygiene to rural Mexico was explicitly dubbed a "health dictatorship" and justified (via stereotypical images of the backward, lazy, and alcoholic poor people of rural Mexico in need of the state's help) as the "only tolerable authoritarianism in a democratic nation" (Aréchiga Córdoba 2005, 119).

5. It is interesting to note that hospitals first took hold in the Americas largely in Mexico. Hernán Cortés built a hospital in the sixteenth century for European Spanish patients to be tended by Spanish physicians after the Mexico–Tenochtitlan Conquest (this hospital is still in operation in Mexico City), and many other hospitals catering to Indigenous, mulattoes, and other marginalized groups followed across the country, generally focusing on providing general social services and spiritual salvation, though some also had medical practitioners on staff (Ayala-García 2014). Early hospitals across the Americas reflected both the desire to convert Indigenous populations to Christianity and the need to treat patients inflicted with imported European diseases for which local healers were not prepared (Wesp 2017).

6. Both IMSS and ISSSTE came out of nationally organized labor movements, though Mexico did turn to the International Labor Organization (ILO) for help in establishing how contributions and benefits would work, a move that tied Mexican social health insurance to globally determined norms (Dion 2008).

7. The hospital has gone through multiple iterations. Early hospitals went from initially serving as places for the poor and destitute to seek shelter or spiritual salvation to spaces to segregate the contagious to military rehabilitation centers to, by the eighteenth century, institutions increasingly focused on curing patients, teaching medical professionals, and conducting medical research (Risse 1999).

8. While more women did attend prenatal visits and more SBAs were trained, neither of these reached the targets set forth by the Millennium Development Goals, and a quarter of women in developing countries still give birth with a relative or alone (Lane and Garrod 2016).

9. During post-revolutionary times, the education of rural Mexican populations emphasized hygiene education, which was seen as equally important to math or geography and which was largely tied to the broader state project of modernization (Aréchiga Córdoba 2005).

10. If the patient wanted a water birth, this could cost double; in addition, if the woman had to have a cesarean section, she could incur much more costs. For this reason, Doña Guadalupe told me that she had begun to see more patients go to CASA for their prenatal care, because they liked how they were treated there, then go to the public hospital for the birth itself, to avoid CASA's birth fees.

11. While LEOs did have less evidence-based training in the past, obstetric nursing programs have increased their adherence to evidence-based practices in recent years, after changing their curricula to specifically address this gap (Atkin et al. 2019).

12. Nurses in Mexico have historically had less power in the health-care system than doctors, owing in part to their degree and status and in part to (real or perceived) class differences; this situation has changed somewhat more recently, as nurses gain higher educational degrees (Squires and Juarez 2012).

13. For this survey, thirty-eight midwifery participants responded, and most gave multiple answers. Twenty-eight were from CASA, and ten were from Mujeres Aliadas. While the CASA students were asked to state which semester they were in within the three-year program, the Mujeres Aliadas students are shown here as one group, because they were all part of the first (and only) cohort of students, finishing their first year of studies.

14. At the time of writing this, CASA's school website announced that it was not taking more students but rather was creating a bachelor's degree in midwifery program.

CHAPTER 2

1. See the Introduction for a discussion about the role of foreign NGOs and for a reminder about the differences between the three schools.

2. The majority of countries in attendance at Beijing's Fourth World Conference on Women the following year "agreed that without the most basic rights for women within the family and society—most of all the right to decide, jointly or alone if necessary, on the number of children they were prepared to bear, or that their health could sustain—meaningful and rapid strides in public health, education, the protection of the environment, and economic development would lag at best and be impossible at worst" (Crossette 2005, 71).

3. See Givaudan et al. (2008) for details of the study and its findings.

CHAPTER 3

1. A common practice in Mexico is to manually remove the placenta and clean out the uterus after birth to prevent infection. Studies indicate that this is unnecessary and can possibly introduce infection: the placenta is usually delivered naturally without intervention shortly after birth, and if it can be determined to be intact upon delivery the uterus need not be manually

cleaned out (Epperly, Fogarty, and Hodges 1989; Alvirde Alvaro and Rodriguez Anguiniga 2009).
2. Indeed, the Mexican reproductive rights NGO, Grupo de Información en Reproducción Elegida (GIRE), took up her case with the government of Oaxaca, claiming that the baby's human rights had been violated; the state agreed to build more delivery rooms to prevent such situations in the future, though by 2015 they had yet to follow through with the construction (GIRE 2015).
3. These programs include the Instituto Mexicano del Seguro Social (IMSS), Instituto de Seguridad y Servicios Sociales de los Trabajadores del Estado (ISSSTE), Petróleos Mexicanos (PEMEX), Secretaría de la Defensa Nacional (SEDENA), and Secretaría de Marina (MARINA).
4. For a comparative analysis of Mexican midwives' professional journeys and relationships with the state, including more details about Julieta's story, see Dixon, El Kotni, and Miranda (2019).

CHAPTER 4

This chapter is derived in part from my article published in *Medical Anthropology Quarterly* in 2015, "Obstetrics in a Time of Violence: Mexican Midwives Critique Routine Hospital Practices," copyright John Wiley and Sons, available online at doi.org/10.1111/maq.12174 (Zacher Dixon 2015). Three of the figures in this chapter (5, 6, and 7) were previously published in *Medical Anthropology* in 2020 in my article "Making Women into Protagonists: Midwives Reimagine the Mexican Childbirth Narrative," copyright Taylor and Francis (Dixon 2020).

1. Arachu Castro's (2004) work reveals that alarming patterns of forced sterilization or IUD insertion immediately postpartum in Mexico are linked to doctors' assumptions that women will not return for follow-up contraceptive counseling and also to attempts on a national level to integrate childbirth and contraceptive services.
2. Despite Ana's concerns, studies have shown that postpartum insertion of an IUD immediately following delivery of the placenta or after a cesarean section can be a safe and practical strategy (even if the risk of expulsion of the device is higher), if and when informed consent is obtained (Cwiak and Cordes 2018).
3. All drawings reproduced here are published with permission of the students who drew them.
4. See (Smith-Oka 2015) for an analysis of cervical examinations as obstetric violence in Mexico.
5. As with Hannah Arendt's 1963 use of the phrase "the banality of evil," I argue here that certain acts of violence become banal in that they are not done with individual, malevolent intentionality, but rather as part of an ingrained, bureaucratic system that justifies and reproduces them.
6. The World Health Organization has long categorized the routine use of Pitocin and episiotomies as "Practices Which Are Frequently Used Inappropriately" (1997, 123). See El Kotni (2018) for an examination of episiotomies as obstetric violence in Mexico.
7. While the risk of infection by remaining pieces of placenta is real, studies indicate that such manual revision is unnecessary if the placenta can be determined to be intact upon delivery, a determination that can be made with the naked eye in a few moments (Epperly, Fogarty, and Hodges 1989; Alvirde Alvaro and Rodriguez Anguiniga 2009).

CHAPTER 5

1. In the 1970s, traditional midwives and nurses attended 40 percent of births in Mexico (Cragin et al. 2007, 51), while now, 96 percent of births in Mexico are attended by doctors in hospitals (Faget and Capasso 2017, 4).

2. When I learned about this, I thought of Juana, all those years ago in Oaxaca (see Introduction), and her liberal use of Pitocin within an otherwise very non-medical setting.

3. Homeopathic medicine has a long history in Mexico, where it gained popularity in the mid-nineteenth century as a way to take care of health issues at home, especially for the majority of the population who could not afford or access licensed doctors (Hernández Berrones 2017). As such, it became a common and popular option for people to turn to alongside both Western and alternative treatments.

CONCLUSION

This chapter is derived in part from my article "Making Women into Protagonists: Midwives Reimagine the Mexican Childbirth Narrative" published in *Medical Anthropology*, copyright Taylor and Francis, available online at doi.org/10.1080/01459740.2020.1714609 (Dixon 2020).

1. The need for midwives and out of hospital birthing options became even clearer during the 2020 COVID-19 pandemic, as hospitals across Mexico (as elsewhere) became increasingly risky (*Efe*, April 1, 2020).

2. During my observations at CASA's hospital, many patients described leaving the public hospital to come to CASA because of how they were treated or choosing CASA for a birth because of how they had been treated at the hospital in the past.

REFERENCES

Abramowitz, Sharon, and Catherine Panter-Brick. 2015. *Medical Humanitarianism: Ethnographies of Practice*. Philadelphia: University of Pennsylvania Press.

Adams, Vincanne. 2016. *Metrics: What Counts in Global Health*. Edited by Vincanne Adams. Durham and London: Duke University Press.

Aguilar Ortega, Teodoro. 2019. "Desarrollo humano y desigualdad en México." *México y la Cuenca del Pacífico* 8 (22): 121–41.

Alonso, Cristina, and Tania Gerard. 2009. "El parto humanizado como herramienta para la prevención de la mortalidad materna y la mejora de la salud materno-infantil." In *La muerte materna: Acciones y estrategias hacia una maternidad segura*, edited by Graciela Freyermuth and Paola Sesia, 95–100. Mexico City: Centro de Investigaciones y Estudios Superioires en Antropología Social: Comitè Promotor por una Maternidad sin Riesgos en Mexico.

Alvirde Alvaro, Osvaldo, and Gerardo Rodriguez Anguiniga. 2009. "Revisión rutinaria de cavidad uterina en el postparto inmediato." *Archivos de investigación materno-infantil* 1 (2): 58–63.

Aréchiga Córdoba, Ernesto. 2005. "Propaganda higiénica en el México Revolucionario, 1917–1934." *Dynamis: Acta Hispanica ad Medicinae Scientiarumque Historiam Illustrandam* 25: 117–43.

Arendt, Hannah. 1963. *Eichmann in Jerusalem: A Report on the Banality of Evil*. New York: Viking Press.

Arms, Suzanne. 1975. *Immaculate Deception: A New Look at Women and Childbirth in America*. Boston: Houghton Mifflin.

Atkin, Lucille C., Kimberli Keith-Brown, Martha W. Rees, Paola Sesia, Gabriela Blanco, Dolores Coronel, Gilmaro Cuellar, Rebeca Hernández, and Clara Yang. 2019. "Strengthening Midwifery in Mexico: Evaluation of Progress 2015–2018." January 2019 Report to the John D. and Catherine T. MacArthur Foundation.

Atkin, Lucille C., Kimberli Keith-Brown, Martha W. Rees, Paola Sesia, Aítza Calixto, Rebeca Hernández, and Fátima Valdivia. 2017. *Iniciativa de la Fundación Macarthur para promover la partería en méxico: Informe de resultados de la línea de base*. Chicago, IL: MacArthur Foundation

Ayala-García, Marco Antonio. 2014. "The First Ten Hospitals on the American Continent." Hektoen Internationl. hekint.org/2017/02/23/the-first-ten-hospitals-on-the-american-continent.

Baker Opperman, Stephanie. 2012. "Modernization and Rural Health in Mexico: The Care of the Tepalcatep Commission." *Endeavour* 37 (1): 47–55.

Bastien, Alison. 2019. "The Spectrum of Traditions in Childbirth in Mexico." *Midwifery Today*, no. 132. midwiferytoday.com/mt-articles/the-spectrum-of-traditions-in-childbirth-in-mexico.

Benoit, Cecilia, and Robbie Davis-Floyd. 2004. "Becoming a Midwife in Canada: Models of Midwifery Education." In *Reconceiving Midwifery*, edited by Ivy Lynn Bourgeault, Cecilia Benoit, and Robbie Davis-Floyd, 169–86. Montreal and Kingston: McGill-Queen's University Press.

Berry, Nicole M. 2010. *Unsafe Motherhood: Mayan Maternal Mortality and Subjectivity in Post-War Guatemala.* New York: Berghahn Books.

Biehl, João. 2005. *Vita: Life in a Zone of Social Abandonment.* Berkeley: University of California Press.

Biehl, João, and Adriana Petryna. 2013. *When People Come First: Critical Studies in Global Health.* Princeton, NJ: Princeton University Press.

Boddy, Janice. 1998. "Remembering Amal: On Birth and the British in Northern Sudan." In *Pragmatic Women and Body Politics*, edited by Margaret Lock and Patricia A. Kaufert, 28–57. Cambridge: Cambridge University Press.

Bohren, Meghan A., Hedieh Mehrtash, Bukola Fawole, Thae Maung Maung, Mamadou Dioulde Balde, Ernest Maya, Soe Soe Thwin, et al. 2019. "How Women Are Treated during Facility-Based Childbirth in Four Countries: A Cross-Sectional Study with Labour Observations and Community-Based Surveys." *Lancet* 394 (10210): 1750–63. doi.org/10.1016/S0140-6736(19)31992-0.

Bourgois, Philippe. 2010. "Recognizing Invisible Violence: A Thirty-Year Ethnographic Retrospective." In *Global Health in Times of Violence*, edited by Barbara Rylko-Bauer, Linda Whiteford, and Paul Farmer, 17–40. Santa Fe: School for Advanced Research Press.

Bourgois, Philippe, Seth M. Holmes, Kim Sue, and James Quesada. 2017. "Structural Vulnerability: Operationalizing the Concept to Address Health Disparities in Clinical Care." *Academic Medicine* 92 (3): 299–307. doi.org/10.1097/ACM.0000000000001294.

Brink, Susan. 2019. "Why Are Health Care Providers Slapping and Yelling at Mothers During Childbirth?" *Goats and Soda* (blog). National Public Radio, October 14, 2019. www.npr.org/sections/goatsandsoda/2019/10/14/769065385/why-are-midwives-and-nurses-slapping-and-yelling-at-mothers-during-childbirth.

Buse, Kent, and Sarah Hawkes. 2015. "Health in the Sustainable Development Goals: Ready for a Paradigm Shift?" *Globalization and Health* 11 (1): 13. doi.org/10.1186/s12992-015-0098-8.

Caldeira, Teresa. 2002. "Paradox of Police Violence in Democratic Brazil." *Ethnography* 3 (3): 235–63.

Calzada Martinez, Heidy. 2009. "Veracruz, primer estado que tipifica como delito la violencia obstétrica: IVM." *Al Calor Político*, November 28, 2009. www.alcalorpolitico.com/informacion/veracruz-primer-estado-que-tipifica-como-delito-la-violencia-obst-tri-ca-ivm-44406.html.

Carrillo, AM. 1999. "Nacimiento y muerte de una profesión." *Dynamis: Acta Hispanica ad Medicinae Scientiarumque Historiam Illustrandam*, no. 19: 167–90.

Carson, Anna, Cathy Chabot, Devon Greyson, Kate Shannon, Putu Duff, and Jean Shoveller. 2017. "A Narrative Analysis of the Birth Stories of Early-Age Mothers." *Sociology of Health and Illness* 39 (6): 816–31. doi.org/10.1111/1467-9566.12518.

Castañeda Núñez, Imelda. 1988. "Síntesis histórica de la partera en el Valle de México." *Revista de enfermería, Instituto Mexicano del Seguro Social (Mexico)* 1 (1): 35–39.

Castro, Arachu. 2004. *Unhealthy Health Policy: A Critical Anthropological Examination.* Edited by Arachu Castro and Merrill Singer. Walnut Creek, CA: AltaMira Press.

Castro, Roberto. 2014. "Health Care Delivery System: Mexico." In *The Wiley Blackwell Encyclopedia of Health, Illness, Behavior, and Society*, 836–42. Chichester, UK: John Wiley and Sons. doi.org/10.1002/9781118410868.wbehibs101.

Castro, Roberto, Corinne Agustin Peek-Asa, and Agustin Ruiz. 2003. "Violence against Women in Mexico: A Study of Abuse Before and During Pregnancy." *American Journal of Public Health* 93 (7): 1110–16.

Chavoustie, Steven E., Scott Eder, William D. Koltun, Tracey R. Lemon, Caroline Mitchell, Paul Nyirjesy, Jack D. Sobel, Ryan Sobel, and Rachel Villanueva. 2017. "Experts Explore the State of Bacterial Vaginosis and the Unmet Needs Facing Women and Providers." *International Journal of Gynecology & Obstetrics* 137: 107–9. doi.org/10.1002/ijgo.12114.

Choy, Timothy K. 2005. "Articulated Knowledges: Environmental Forms after Universality's Demise." *American Anthropologist* 107 (1): 5–18. doi.org/10.2307/3567668.

_____. 2011. *Ecologies of Comparison: An Ethnography of Endangerment in Hong Kong.* Durham and London: Duke University Press.

Closser, Svea. 2010. *Chasing Polio in Pakistan: Why the World's Largest Public Health Initiative May Fail.* Nashville, TN: Vanderbilt University Press.

Coatecatl, Jaquelin. 2013. "Hospital de Oaxaca obliga a indígena a dar a luz en el pasto." *La razón*, October 5, 2013.

Coerver, Don M., Suzanne B. Pasztor, and Robert Buffington. 2004. *Mexico: An Encyclopedia of Contemporary Culture and History.* Santa Barbara, CA: ABC-CLIO.

Cohen Shabot, S. 2016. "Making Loud Bodies 'Feminine': A Feminist-Phenomenological Analysis of Obstetric Violence." *Human Studies* 39 (2): 231–47.

Cole, Teju. 2012. "The White-Savior Industrial Complex." *Atlantic*, March 12, 2012. www.theatlantic.com/international/archive/2012/03/the-white-savior-industrial-complex/254843.

CONAPO (Consejo Nacional de Población). 2016. *Situación de la salud sexual y reproductiva. República mexicana.* México, D.F. www.gob.mx/conapo.

COPLAMAR. 1983. "Necesidades esenciales en México: Salud, situación y perspectivas al año 2000." *Siglo XXI/COPLAMAR* Mexico.

Cortés, Rubén. 2013. "Parir en el pasto en un país de la OCDE." *La razón*, October 7, 2013.

Cragin, Leslie, Lisa M. DeMaria, Lourdes Campero, and Dilys M. Walker. 2007. "Educating Skilled Birth Attendants in Mexico: Do the Curricula Meet International Confederation of Midwives Standards?" *Reproductive Health Matters* 15 (30): 50–60.

Crossette, Barbara. 2005. "Reproductive Health and the Millennium Development Goals: The Missing Link." *Studies in Family Planning* 36 (1): 71–79.

Cwiak, Carrie, and Sarah Cordes. 2018. "Postpartum Intrauterine Device Placement: A Patient-Friendly Option." *Contraception and Reproductive Medicine* 3: 3. doi.org/10.1186/s40834-018-0057-x.

Dall, Tim. 2018. "2018 Update. The Complexities of Physician Supply and Demand: Projections from 2016 to 2030. Final Report." Association of American Medical Colleges. doi.org/10.13140/RG.2.2.25694.48963.

Daniels, Susannah. 2015. "Raised on My Mother's Love Alone: A Mayan Theater Collective Contests Gender Violence." *American Indian Culture and Research Journal* 39 (4): 93–112. doi.org/10.17953/aicrj.39.4.daniels.

Davis-Floyd, Robbie. 1987. "Obstetric Training as a Rite of Passage." *Medical Anthropology Quarterly* 1 (3): 288–318. doi.org/10.1525/maq.1987.1.3.02a00050.

_____. 2001a. "La Partera Profesional: Articulating Identity and Cultural Space for a New Kind of Midwife in Mexico." *Medical Anthropology* 20 (2–3): 185–243. www.davis-floyd.com/Articles/DF22.pdf.

_____. 2001b. "The Technocratic, Humanistic, and Holistic Paradigms of Childbirth." *International Journal of Gynecology and Obstetrics* 75: 5–23. www.davis-floyd.com.

————. 2005. "Daughters of Time: The Postmodern Midwife." *MIDIRS Midwifery Digest* 15: 32–39.

Davis-Floyd, Robbie, Lesley Barclay, Betty-Anne Daviss, and Jan Tritten. 2009. "Introduction." In *Birth Models That Work*, edited by Robbie E. Davis-Floyd, Lesley Barclay, Jan Tritten, and Betty-Anne Daviss, 1–30. Berkeley: University of California Press.

Davis-Floyd, Robbie, and Joseph Dumit. 1998. "Cyborg Babies: Children of the Third Millenium." In *Cyborg Babies: From Techno-Sex to Techno-Tots*, edited by Robbie Davis-Floyd and Joseph Dumit, 1–20. New York: Routledge.

Davis-Floyd, Robbie, S. L. Pigg, and S. Cosminsky. 2001. "Introduction. Daughters of Time: The Shifting Identities of Contemporary Midwives." *Medical Anthropology* 20 (2–3): 105–39. www.ncbi.nlm.nih.gov/pubmed/11817853.

Davis-Floyd, Robbie, and Carolyn F. Sargent. 1997. *Childbirth and Authoritative Knowledge: Cross-Cultural Perspectives*. Berkeley: University of California Press.

Davis, Dána-Ain. 2019. *Reproductive Injustice: Racism, Pregnancy, and Premature Birth*. New York: New York University Press.

Del Castillo Negrete Rovira, Miguel. 2017. "Income Inequality in Mexico, 2004–2014." *Latin American Policy* 8 (1): 93–113. doi.org/10.1111/lamp.12112.

Diaz Olavarrieta, Claudia, and Julio Sotelo. 1996. "Domestic Violence in Mexico." *JAMA: The Journal of the American Medical Association* 275 (24): 1937–41.

Dion, Michelle. 2008. "International Organizations and Social Insurance in Mexico." *Global Social Policy* 8 (1): 25–44. doi.org/10.1177/1468018107086086.

Dixon, Lydia Zacher. 2019. "Birthing in the Field." In *Mothering from the Field: The Impact of Motherhood on Site-Based Research*, edited by Bahiyyah M. Muhammad and Mélanie-Angela Nueilly, 62–75. New Brunsqick, NJ: Rutgers University Press.

————. 2020. "Making Women into Protagonists: Midwives Reimagine the Mexican Childbirth Narrative." *Medical Anthropology*. January 23, 2020. doi.org/10.1080/01459740.2020.1714609.

Dixon, Lydia Zacher, Mounia El Kotni, and Veronica Miranda. 2019. "A Tale of Three Midwives: Inconsistent Policies and the Marginalization of Midwifery in Mexico." *Journal of Latin American and Caribbean Anthropology* 24 (2): 351–69. doi.org/10.1111/jlca.12384.

Dixon, Lydia Zacher, Vania Smith-Oka, and Mounia El Kotni. 2019. "Teaching about Childbirth in Mexico: Working across Birth Models." In *Birth in Eight Cultures*, edited by Robbie Davis-Floyd and Melissa Cheyney, 17–48. Long Grove, IL: Waveland Press.

DONA. n.d. "What Is a Doula?" Accessed January 8, 2020. www.dona.org/what-is-a-doula/.

Doubova, Svetlana V., Sebastián García-Saiso, Ricardo Pérez-Cuevas, Odet Sarabia-González, Paulina Pacheco-Estrello, Claudia Infante-Castañeda, Carmen Santamaría, Laura del Pilar Torres-Arreola, and Hannah H. Leslie. 2018. "Quality Governance in a Pluralistic Health System: Mexican Experience and Challenges." *Lancet Global Health* 6 (11): e1149–52. doi.org/10.1016/S2214-109X(18)30321-8.

Doubova, Svetlana V., Sebastián García-Saisó, Ricardo Pérez-Cuevas, Odet Sarabia-González, Paulina Pacheco-Estrello, Hannah H. Leslie, Carmen Santamaría, Laura del Pilar Torres-Arreola, and Claudia Infante-Castañeda. 2018. "Barriers and Opportunities to Improve the Foundations for High-Quality Healthcare in the Mexican Health System." *Health Policy and Planning* 33 (10): 1073–82. doi.org/10.1093/heapol/czy098.

Duncan, Whitney L. 2017. "Psicoeducación in the Land of Magical Thoughts: Culture and Mental-Health Practice in a Changing Oaxaca." *American Ethnologist* 44 (1): 36–51. doi.org/10.1111/amet.12424.

Eckstein, Susan, ed. 2001. *Power and Popular Protest: Latin American Social Movements*. Los Angeles: University of California Press.

Efe. 2020. "El miedo de contraer la COVID-19 lleva a mexicanas a dar a luz en sus casas." April 1, 2020. www.efe.com/efe/usa/mexico/el-miedo-de-contraer-la-covid-19-lleva-a-mexicanas-dar-luz-en-sus-casas/50000100-4210955

El Kotni, Mounia. 2016. "'Porque tienen mucho derecho': Parteras, Biomedical Training and the Vernacularization of Human Rights in Chiapas." PhD diss., State University of New York at Albany.

————. 2018. "Between Cut and Consent: Indigenous Women's Experiences of Obstetric Violence in Mexico." *American Indian Culture and Research Journal* 42 (4): 21–41. doi. org/10.17953/aicrj.42.4.elkotni.

————. 2019. "Regulating Traditional Mexican Midwifery: Practices of Control, Strategies of Resistance." *Medical Anthropology* 38 (2): 137–51. doi.org/10.1080/01459740.2018.1539974.

Elgar, Richard. 2014. "Women's Rights in Transition: The Collision of Feminist Interest Groups, Religion and Non-Governmental Organizations in Three Latin American Countries." *Journal of Public Affairs* 14 (3–4): 359–68. doi.org/10.1002/pa.430.

Elsubai, Ibrahim, and Tamer Aboushanab. 2017. "History of Cupping (Hijama): A Narrative Review of Literature." *Journal of Integrative Medicine* 15 (3): 172–81.

Epperly, T. D., J. P. Fogarty, and S. G. Hodges. 1989. "Efficacy of Routine Postpartum Uterine Exploration and Manual Sponge Curettage." *Journal of Family Practice* 28 (2): 172–76. www.ncbi.nlm.nih.gov/pubmed/2783726.

Faget, María, and Ariadna Capasso. 2017. "Partería en México." Management Sciences for Health. Mexico City, Mexico. www.msh.org/sites/msh.org/files/parteria_en_mexico_midwifery_in_mexico_spanish.pdf.

Fajardo-Ortiz, Guillermo. 2008. "Inicios de la atención médica en el Instituto Mexicano del Seguro Social en Oaxaca." *Boletín mexicano de historia y filosofía de la medicina* 11 (1): 26–28.

Faneite, Josmery, Alejandra Feo, and Judith Toro Merlo. 2012. "Grado de conocimiento de violencia obstétrica por el personal de salud." *Revista de obstetricia y ginecología de Venezuela* 72 (1): 4–12.

Farmer, Paul. 1996. "On Suffering and Structural Violence: A View from Below." *Daedalus* 125, no. 1 (Winter): 261–83.

————. 2004. "Anthropology of Structural Violence." *Current Anthropology* 45 (3): 305–25.

Fassin, Didier. 2009. "A Violence of History: Accounting for AIDS in Post-Apartheid South Africa." In *Global Health in Times of Violence*, edited by Barbara Rylko-Bauer, Linda Whiteford, and Paul Farmer, 113–35. Santa Fe: School for Advanced Research Press.

Fernandez Canton, Sonia B., Gonzalo Gutierrez Trujillo, and Ricardo Viguri Uribe. 2012. "Maternal Mortality and Abortion in Mexico." *Boletín médico del Hospital Infantil de México* 69 (1): 73–76.

Finkler, Kaja. 1994. *Women in Pain: Gender and Morbidity in Mexico*. Philadelphia: University of Pennsylvania Press.

Flores, Francisco A. 1886. *Historia de la medicina en México desde la epoca de los indios hasta la presente*. Mexico: Oficina tip. de la Secretaría de fomento. archive.org/details/historiadelamedio3unse/page/592.

Foucault, Michel. 1973. *The Birth of the Clinic: An Archaeology of Medical Perception*. New York: Vintage.

Freyermuth, Graciela, and Paola Sesia. 2009. *La muerte materna: Acciones y estrategias hacia una maternidad segura*. Mexico City, Mexico: Comité Promotor por una Maternidad sin Riesgos.

Galtung, Johan. 1969. "Violence, Peace and Peace Research." *Journal of Peace Research* 6 (3): 167–91.

———. 1990. "Cultural Violence." *Journal of Peace Research* 27 (3): 291–305.

Garcia, Francisco, Elena Mendez de Galaz, Susie Baldwin, Mary Papenfuss, Anna R. Giuliano, Kenneth Hatch, and John Davis. 2003. "Factors That Affect the Quality of Cytologic Cervical Cancer Screening along the Mexico-United States Border." *American Journal of Obstetrics and Gynecology* 189 (2): 467–72. doi.org/10.1067/S0002-9378(03)00490-3.

Gaskin, Ina May. 2002. *Spiritual Midwifery*. Summertown, TN: Book Publishing Company.

Ginsburg, Faye, and Rayna Rapp. 1991. "The Politics of Reproduction." *Annual Review of Anthropology* 20 (January): 311–43. doi.org/10.1146/annurev.an.20.100191.001523.

———, eds. 1995. *Conceiving the New World Order: The Global Politics of Reproduction*. Berkeley: University of California Press.

GIRE (Grupo de Información en Reproducción Elegida). 2012. *20 años por todas las mujeres*. Mexico City: Grupo de Información en Reproducción Elegida. gire.org.mx/wp-content/uploads/2016/07/20aniosportodas.pdf.

———. 2015. *Obstetric Violence: A Human Rights Approach*. Mexico City: Grupo de Información en Reproducción Elegida. gire.org.mx/en/informes/obstetric-violence-a-human-rights-approach-2015.

Givaudan, Martha, Iwin Leenen, Susan Pick, Andrea Angulo, and Ype H. Poortinga. 2008. "Enhancement of Underused Cervical Cancer Prevention Services in Rural Oaxaca, Mexico." *Revista panamericana de salud pública* 23 (2): 135–43. doi.org/10.1590/S1020-49892008000200015.

Goldstein, Donna. 2007. "Life or Profit?: Structural Violence, Moral Psychology and Pharmaceutical Politics." *Anthropology in Action* 14 (3): 44–58.

Gómez Dantés, Octavio, Sergio Sesma, Victor M. Becerril, Felicia M. Knaul, Hector Arreola, and Julio Frenk. 2011. "Sistema de salud de Mexico." *Salud publica de Mexico* 53 (2): S2220–32.

González, Luis. 1981. *Historia de la revolución mexicana, 1934-1940: Los días del Presidente Cárdenas*. Mexico City, Mexico: El Colegio de México.

Good, Byron J., and Mary-Jo Del Vecchio Good. 1993. "Learning Medicine: The Construction of Medical Knowledge at Harvard Medical School." In *Knowledge, Power and Practice: The Anthropology of Medicine and Everyday Life*, edited by Shirley Lindenbaum and Margaret Lock, 81–107. Los Angeles: University of California Press.

Goode, Keisha La'Nesha. 2014. "Birthing, Blackness, and the Body: Black Midwives and Experiential Continuities of Institutional Racism." PhD diss., City University of New York. academicworks.cuny.edu/gc_etds/423.

Guerra-Reyes, Lucia. 2019. *Changing Birth in the Andes: Culture, Policy, and Safe Motherhood in Peru*. Nashville, TN: Vanderbilt University Press.

Guerra Falcon, Aida. 2009. *Medicina traditional: Doña Queta y el legado de los habitantes de las nubes*. Oaxaca City, Mexico: Hamalgama Editorial.

Gurr, Barbara. 2014. *Reproductive Justice: The Politics of Health Care for Native American Women*. New Brunsqick, NJ: Rutgers University Press. doi.org/10.5860/choice.189050.

Gutmann, Matthew. 2011. "Planning Men out of Family Planning: A Case Study from Mexico." In *Reproduction, Globalization and the State: New Theoretical and Ethnographic Perspectives*, edited by Carole H. Browner and Carolyn F. Sargent, 53–67. Durham, NC: Duke University Press.

Haraway, Donna. 1988. "Situated Knowledges: The Science Question in Feminism and the Privilege of Partial Perspective." *Feminist Studies* 14 (3): 575–99.

Harding, Sandra. 1998. *Is Science Multicultural? Postcolonialisms, Feminisms, and Epistemologies*. Bloomington, IN: Indiana University Press.

Hausman, Bernice L. 2005. "Risky Business: Framing Childbirth in Hospital Settings." *Journal of Medical Humanities* 26 (1): 23–38.

Heredia-Pi, Ileana, Edson Servan-Mori, Blair G. Darney, Hortensia Reyes-Morales, and Rafael Lozano. 2016. "Measuring the Adequacy of Antenatal Health Care: A National Cross-Sectional Study in Mexico." *Bulletin of the World Health Organization* 94 (6). www.ncbi.nlm.nih.gov/pmc/articles/PMC4890208/.

Hernández Berrones, Jethro. 2017. "Homeopathy 'for Mexicans': Medical Popularisation, Commercial Endeavours, and Patients' Choice in the Mexican Medical Marketplace, 1853-1872." *Medical History* 61 (4): 568–89. doi.org/10.1017/mdh.2017.59.

Hobbs, Amy J., Ann-Beth Moller, Alisa Kachikis, Liliana Carvajal-Aguirre, Lale Say, and Doris Chou. 2019. "Scoping Review to Identify and Map the Health Personnel Considered Skilled Birth Attendants in Low-and-Middle Income Countries from 2000–2015." Edited by Zohra S Lassi. *PLOS ONE* 14 (2): e0211576. doi.org/10.1371/journal.pone.0211576.

Hogan, Margaret C., Biani Saavedra-Avendano, Blair G. Darney, Luis M. Torres-Palacios, Ana L. Rhenals-Osorio, Bertha L. Vázquez Sierra, Patricia N. Soliz-Sánchez, Emmanuela Gakidou, and Rafael Lozano. 2016. "Reclassification des causes obstétricales de décès au Mexique: Une étude transversale répétée." *Bulletin of the World Health Organization* 94 (5): 362-369B. doi.org/10.2471/BLT.15.163360.

Hunt, Paul, and Judith Bueno De Mesquita. 2007. *Reducing Maternal Mortality: The Contribution of the Right to the Highest Attainable Standard of Health*. Essex, UK: University of Essex Human Rights Centre. www.unfpa.org/sites/default/files/pub-pdf/reducing_mm.pdf.

INEGI (Instituto Nacional de Estadística y Geografía). 2015. "Encuesta Nacional de La Dinámica Demográfica ENADID 2014 Principales Resultados." www.beta.inegi.org.mx/contenidos/programas/enadid/2014/doc/resultados_enadid14.pdf.

————. 2018. "Estadísticas a propósito del día internacional de la eliminación de la violencia contra la mujer: Datos nacionales." www.inegi.org.mx/contenidos/saladeprensa/aproposito/2018/violencia2018_Nal.pdf.

INPI (Instituto Nacional de los Pueblos Indígenas). 2018. "Mujeres indígenas, datos estadísticos en el México actual." www.gob.mx/inpi/es/articulos/mujeres-indigenas-datos-estadisticos-en-el-mexico-actual.

Jeffery, Roger, and Patricia M. Jeffery. 1993. "Traditional Birth Attendants in Rural North India: The Social Organization of Childbearing." In *Knowledge, Power and Practice: The Anthropology of Medicine and Everyday Life*, edited by Shirley Lindenbaum and Margaret Lock, 7–31. Berkeley: University of California Press.

Jesús-García, Abraham de, Sergio Paredes-Solís, Geovani Valtierra-Gil, Felipe Rene Serrano-de los Santos, Belén Madeline Sánchez-Gervacio, Robert J. Ledogar, Neil Andersson, and Anne Cockcroft. 2018. "Associations with Perineal Trauma during Childbirth at Home and in Health Facilities in Indigenous Municipalities in Southern Mexico: A Cross-Sectional Cluster Survey." *BMC Pregnancy and Childbirth* 18 (1): 198. doi.org/10.1186/s12884-018-1836-8.

Jewkes, Rachel, and Loveday Penn-Kekana. 2015. "Mistreatment of Women in Childbirth: Time for Action on This Important Dimension of Violence against Women." *PLOS Medicine* 12 (6): e1001849. doi.org/10.1371/journal.pmed.1001849.

Jiménez, Arturo. 2012. "Presentan una obra sobre la partería y el parto humanizado." *La jornada*, June 12, 2012. www.jornada.com.mx/2012/06/04/cultura/a09n1cul.

Jordan, Brigitte. 1978. *Birth in Four Cultures: A Crosscultural Investigation of Childbirth in Yucatan, Holland, Sweden, and the United States.* Prospect Heights, IL: Waveland Press.

———. 1997. "Authoritative Knowledge and Its Construction." In *Childbirth and Authoritative Knowledge,* edited by Carolyn F. Sargent and Robbie Davis-Floyd, 55–79. Los Angeles: University of California Press.

Justice, Judith. 1987. "The Bureaucratic Context of International Health: A Social Scientist's View." *Social Science and Medicine* 25 (12): 1301–6. doi.org/10.1016/0277-9536(87)90128-6.

———. 1989. *Policies, Plans, and People: Foreign Aid and Health Development.* Berkeley, CA: University of California Press.

Katz Rothman, Barbara. 1991. *In Labor: Women and Power in the Birthplace.* New York: Norton.

Kaufert, Patricia, and John O'Neil. 1993. "Analysis of a Dialogue on Risks in Childbirth: Clinicians, Epidemiologists, and Inuit Women." In *Knowledge, Power and Practice: The Anthropology of Medicine and Everyday Life,* edited by Shirley Lindenbaum and Margaret Lock, 32–54. Berkeley: University of California Press.

Khokhar, Tariq, and Umar Serajuddin. 2015. "Should We Continue to Use the Term 'Developing World'?" World Bank Data Blog. 2015. blogs.worldbank.org/opendata/should-we-continue-use-term-developing-world.

Knaul, Felicia Marie, and Julio Frenk. 2005. "Health Insurance In Mexico: Achieving Universal Coverage Through Structural Reform." *Health Affairs* 24 (6): 1467–76. doi.org/10.1377/hlthaff.24.6.1467.

Krieger, Nancy. 2005. "Embodiment: A Conceptual Glossary for Epidemiology." *Journal of Epidemiological Community Health* 59: 350–55.

La prensa. 2013. "Clinica cobra a mujer tras dar a luz en cesped." *La prensa,* October 8, 2013.

Lakoff, Andrew. 2010. "Two Regimes of Global Health." *Humanity* 1 (1): 59–79. doi.org/10.1353/hum.2010.0001.

Lane, Karen, and Jayne Garrod. 2016. "The Return of the Traditional Birth Attendant." *Journal of Global Health* 6 (2). doi.org/10.7189/jogh.06.020302.

Langwick, Stacey A. 2008. "Articulate(d) Bodies: Traditional Medicine in a Tanzanian Hospital." *American Ethnologist* 35: 428–39.

——— 2011. *Bodies, Politics and African Healing: The Matter of Maladies in Tanzania.* Bloomington, IN: Indiana University Press.

Lazcano-Ponce, Eduardo Cesar, Patricia Alonso de Ruiz, Lizbeth Lopez-Carrillo, Maria Eugenia Vazquez-Manriquez, and Mauricio Hernandez-Avila. 1994. "Quality Control Study on Negative Gynecological Cytology in Mexico." *Diagnostic Cytopathology* 10 (1): 10–14. doi.org/10.1002/dc.2840100104.

León, Nicolas. 1910. *La obstetricia en México. Notas bibliográficas, etnicas, históricas, documentarias y críticas, de los orígenes históricos hasta el año 1910.* Mexico City: Tip. de la. Vda. de F. Diaz de Leon, Sucrs.

Livingston, Julie. 2012. *Improvising Medicine: An African Oncology Ward in an Emerging Cancer Epidemic.* Durham and London: Duke University Press.

Lock, Margaret, and Vinh-Kim Nguyen. 2010. *An Anthropology of Biomedicine.* Oxford: Wiley-Blackwell.

Lopez, Laureen M., Alissa Bernholc, David Hubacher, Gretchen Stuart, and Huib A. A. M. Van Vliet. 2015. "Immediate Postpartum Insertion of Intrauterine Device for Contraception." *Cochrane Database of Systematic Reviews,* June 26, 2015. doi.org/10.1002/14651858. CD003036.pub3.

MacDonald, Margaret. 2007. *At Work in the Field of Birth: Midwifery Narratives of Nature, Tradition, and Home.* Nashville, TN: Vanderbilt University Press.

MacDorman, Marian F., Eugene Declercq, Howard Cabral, and Christine Morton. 2016. "Recent Increases in the U.S. Maternal Mortality Rate: Disentangling Trends From Measurement Issues." *Obstetrics and Gynecology* 128 (3): 447–55. doi.org/10.1097/AOG.0000000000001556.

Maes, Kenneth, Svea Closser, Ethan Vorel, and Yihenew Tesfaye. 2015. "A Women's Development Army: Narratives of Community Health Worker Investment and Empowerment in Rural Ethiopia." *Studies in Comparative International Development* 50 (4): 455–78. doi.org/10.1007/s12116-015-9197-z.

Maine, Deborah, Murat Z. Akalin, Victoria M. Ward, and Angela Kamara. 1997. *The Design and Evaluation of Maternal Mortality Programs*. New York: Center for Population and Family Health School of Public Health, Columbia University. www.publichealth.columbia.edu/sites/default/files/pdf/designevalmm-en.pdf.

Martin, Emily. 1987. *The Woman in the Body: A Cultural Analysis of Reproduction*. Boston: Beacon Press.

Mayhew, Susannah, Megan Douthwaite, and Michael Hammer. 2006. "Balancing Protection and Pragmatism: A Framework for NGO Accountability in Rights-Based Approaches." *Health and Human Rights* 9 (2): 180–206. www.ncbi.nlm.nih.gov/pubmed/17265760.

McCarthy, J., and D. Maine. 1992. "A Framework for Analyzing the Determinants of Maternal Mortality." *Studies in Family Planning* 23: 23–33.

Mills, Lisa. 2010. "Citizenship, Reproductive Rights, and Maternal Health in Mexico." *Canadian Journal of Development Studies / Revue canadienne d'études du développement* 31 (3–4): 417–38. doi.org/10.1080/02255189.2010.3673728.

Mills, Lisa, and Robbie Davis-Floyd. 2009. "The CASA Hospital and Professional Midwifery School: An Education and Practice Model That Works." In *Birth Models That Work*, edited by Robbie E. Davis-Floyd, Lesley Barclay, Jan Tritten, and Betty-Anne Daviss, 305–36. Berkeley: University of California Press.

Mino, Fernando. 2012. "Parir con dolor: La violencia obstétrica en los servicios de salud." *La jornada*, April 5, 2012. www.jornada.unam.mx/2012/04/05/ls-central.html.

Miranda, Veronica. 2015. "Lingering Discourses from Yucatán's Past: Political Ecologies of Birth in Rural Yucatán." In *The Maya of the Cochuah Region: Archaeological and Ethnographic Perspectives on the Northern Lowlands*, edited by Justine M. Shaw, 235–56. Albuquerque: University of New Mexico Press.

————. 2017. "Reproducing Childbirth: Negotiated Maternal Health Practices in Rural Yucatán." PhD diss., University of Kentucky. doi.org/10.13023/ETD.2017.247.

Mitford, Jessica. 1992. *The American Way of Birth*. New York: Dutton.

Moloney, Anistasia. 2019. "As Venezuela's Healthcare Collapses, Pregnant Women, Girls Bear Brunt of Crisis." *Reuters*, July 8, 2019. www.reuters.com/article/us-venezuela-health-women/as-venezuelas-healthcare-collapses-pregnant-women-girls-bear-brunt-of-crisis-idUSKCN1U32AS.

Monroy-Gómez-Franco, Luis A., Roberto Vélez Grajales, and Gastón Yalonetzky. 2018. *Layers of Inequality: Social Mobility, Inequality of Opportunity and Skin Colour in Mexico*. Mexico City, Mexico: Centro de Estudios Espinoso Yglesias. ceey.org.mx/wp-content/uploads/2018/12/03-MGF-Velez-Yalonetzky-2018.pdf.

Morgan, Lynn M., and Elizabeth F. S. Roberts. 2012. "Reproductive Governance in Latin America." *Anthropology and Medicine* 19 (2): 241–54. doi.org/10.1080/13648470.2012.675046.

Murphy, Michelle. 2017. "Alterlife and Decolonial Chemical Relations." *Cultural Anthropology* 32 (4): 494–503. doi.org/10.14506/ca32.4.02.

Murray de López, Jenna. 2015. "Conflict and Reproductive Health in Urban Chiapas: Disappearing the Partera Empírica." *Anthropology Matters* 16 (1).

Narro Robles, José, and David Moctezuma Navarro. 2012. "Analfabetismo en México: Una deuda social." *Realidad, datos y espacio: Revista internacional de estadística y geografía* 3 (1): 5–17.

Nichter, Mark, and Melanie Angel Medeiros. 2015. "Critical Anthropology for Global Health: What Can It Contribute to Critical Health Psychology?" In *Critical Health Psychology*, edited by Michael Murray, 2nd ed., 291–397. New York: Palgrave Macmillan.

Nunzio, Marco Di. 2018. "Anthropology of Infrastructure." London: LSE Cities, London School of Economics and Political Science. lsecities.net/wpcontent/uploads/2018/09/Governing-Infrastructure-Interfaces_Anthropology-of-infrastrcuture_MarcoDiNunzio.pdf

OECD (Organisation for Economic Cooperation and Development). 2016. "OECD Reviews of Health Systems MEXICO Contents." *OECD iLibrary,* January 6, 2016. doi.org/10.1787/9789264230491-en.

OMM (Observatorio de Mortalidad Materna). 2019. "Boletines de mortalidad materna 2019." 2019. www.omm.org.mx/index.php/indicadores-nacionales/boletines-de-mortalidad-materna/boletines-de-mortalidad-materna-2019.

Oni-Orisan, Adeola. 2016. "The Obligation to Count: The Politics of Monitoring Maternal Mortality in Nigeria." In *Metrics: What Counts in Global Health*, edited by Vincanne Adams, 82–103. Durham and London: Duke University Press.

Page, L. 2001. "The Humanization of Birth." *International Journal of Gynecology and Obstetrics* 75 (1): S55–58.

Pascali-Bonaro, Debra, dir. 2008. *Orgasmic Birth: The Best Kept Secret*. Westlake Village, CA: Seedsman Group. DVD, 85 min. www.orgasmicbirth.com

Paz, Octavio. 1994. *The Labyrinth of Solitude and Other Stories*. New York: Grove Press.

Penyak, Lee M. 2003. "Obstetrics and the Emergence of Women in Mexico's Medical Establishment." *The Americas* 60 (1): 59–85.

Pérez D'Gregorio, Rogelio. 2010. "Obstetric Violence: A New Legal Term Introduced in Venezuela." *International Journal of Gynecology and Obstetrics* 111 (3): 201–2.

Peterson, Gayle. 1984. *Birthing Normally: A Personal Growth Approach to Childbirth*. Berkeley, CA: Shadow and Light.

Pick, Susan, Martha Givaudan, and Michael R. Reich. 2008. "NGO—Government Partnerships for Scaling Up: Sexuality Education in Mexico." *Development in Practice* 18 (2): 164–75. doi.org/10.1080/09614520801897279.

Pigg, Stacy Leigh. 1997. "Authority in Translation: Finding, Knowing, Naming, and Training 'Traditional Birth Attendants' in Nepal." In *Childbirth and Authoritative Knowledge*, edited by Robbie Davis-Floyd and Carolyn Sargent, 233–62. Los Angeles: University of California Press.

Powell, T. G. 1968. "Mexican Intellectuals and the Indian Question, 1876–1911." *Hispanic American Historical Review* 48 (1): 19. doi.org/10.2307/2511398.

Priego, Natalia. 2008. "Symbolism, Solitude and Modernity: Science and Scientists in Porfirian Mexico." *Historia, ciencias, saude—Manguinhos* 15, no. 2 (April/June): 473–85. doi.org/10.1590/S0104-59702008000200016.

Puyana, Alicia, and Sandra Murillo. 2012. "Trade Policies and Ethnic Inequalities in Mexico." *European Journal of Development Research* 24 (5): 706–34. doi.org/10.1057/ejdr.2012.23.

Reyes-Foster, Beatriz M. 2018. "Psychiatric Encounters: Madness and Modernity in Yucatan." New Brunsqick, NJ: Rutgers University Press. muse.jhu.edu/book/63184.

Rich, Adrienne. 1976. *Of Woman Born: Motherhood as Experience and Institution*. New York: Norton.

Richard, Analiese M. 2009. "Mediating Dilemmas: Local NGOs and Rural Development in Neoliberal Mexico." *PoLAR: Political and Legal Anthropology Review* 32 (2): 166–94. doi. org/10.1111/j.1555-2934.2009.01040.x.

Riessman, C. K. 1983. "Women and Medicalization." *Social Policy* 14 (1): 3–18.

Rignall, Karen E. 2019. "Is Rurality a Form of Gender-Based Violence in Morocco?" *Journal of Applied Language and Culture Studies*, no. 2: 15–33.

Risse, Guenter B. 1999. *Mending Bodies, Saving Souls: A History of Hospitals*. New York: Oxford University Press.

Robinson, Nuriya, Cynthia Stoffel, and Sadia Haider. 2015. "Global Women's Health Is More than Maternal Health: A Review of Gynecology Care Needs in Low-Resource Settings." *Obstetrical and Gynecological Survey* 70 (3): 211–22. doi.org/10.1097/OGX.0000000000000166.

Rodgers, Dennis, and Bruce O'Neill. 2012. "Infrastructural Violence: Introduction to the Special Issue." *Ethnography* 13 (4): 401–12. doi.org/10.1177/1466138111435738.

Rodríguez-Aguilar, Román. 2018. "Maternal Mortality in Mexico, beyond Millennial Development Objectives: An Age-Period-Cohort Model." Edited by Massimo Ciccozzi. *PLOS ONE* 13 (3): e0194607. doi.org/10.1371/journal.pone.0194607.

Roldán, José, Marsela Álvarez, María Carrasco, Noé Guarneros, José Ledesma, Mario Cuchillo-Hilario, and Adolfo Chávez. 2017. "Marginalization and Health Service Coverage among Indigenous, Rural, and Urban Populations: A Public Health Problem in Mexico." *Rural and Remote Health* 17 (4). doi.org/10.22605/RRH3948.

Ronsmans, Carine, and Wendy J. Graham. 2006. "Maternal Mortality: Who, When, Where, and Why." *Lancet* 368 (9542): 1189–1200. doi.org/10.1016/S0140-6736(06)69380-X.

Rubin, Sarah E. 2018. "'The Inimba It Cuts': A Reconsideration of Mother Love in the Context of Poverty." *Ethos* 46 (3): 330–50. doi.org/10.1111/etho.12210.

Rylko-Bauer, Barbara, Linda Whiteford, and Paul Farmer. 2009. *Global Health in Times of Violence*. Santa Fe: School for Advanced Research Press.

Sachse-Aguilera, Matthias, and Omar Calvo-Aguilar. 2013. "Indicaciones de la revisión manual de la cavidad uterina durante la tercera etapa de trabajo de parto: Revisión de la evidencia." *Revista CONAMED* 18, no. 1 (January–March): 31–36.

Sadler, Michelle, Mário J. D. S. Santos, Dolores Ruiz-Berdún, Gonzalo Leiva Rojas, Elena Skoko, Patricia Gillen, and Jette A. Clausen. 2016. "Moving beyond Disrespect and Abuse: Addressing the Structural Dimensions of Obstetric Violence." *Reproductive Health Matters* 24 (47): 47–55. doi.org/10.1016/j.rhm.2016.04.002.

Sánchez Inzunza, Alejandra. 2020. "Parir en México es un acto de resistencia." *Washington Post*, January 13, 2020.

Sankaranarayanan, Rengaswamy, Atul Madhukar Budukh, and Rajamanickam Rajkumar. 2001. "Effective Screening Programmes for Cervical Cancer in Low- and Middle-Income Developing Countries." World Health Organization. *Bulletin of the World Health Organization* 79: 954.

Sarmiento, Iván, Sergio Paredes-Solís, Neil Andersson, and Anne Cockcroft. 2018. "Safe Birth and Cultural Safety in Southern Mexico: Study Protocol for a Randomised Controlled Trial." *Trials* 19 (1): 354. doi.org/10.1186/s13063-018-2712-6.

Say, Lale, Doris Chou, Alison Gemmill, Özge Tunçalp, Ann Beth Moller, Jane Daniels, A. Metin Gülmezoglu, Marleen Temmerman, and Leontine Alkema. 2014. "Global Causes of Maternal Death: A WHO Systematic Analysis." *Lancet Global Health* 2 (6). doi.org/10.1016/S2214-109X(14)70227-X.

Schaefer Muñoz, Sara. 2017. "Venezuelan Women in Labor Cross to Colom-
bia to Give Birth." *Wall Street Journal*, March 23, 2017. www.wsj.com/articles/
venezuelan-women-in-labor-cross-to-colombia-to-give-birth-1490261402.

Scheper-Hughes, Nancy. 1992. *Death without Weeping: The Violence of Everyday Life in Brazil.*
Berkeley: University of California Press.

Schuller, Mark. 2012. *Killing with Kindness: Haiti, International Aid, and NGOs.* New Bruns-
wick, NJ: Rutgers University Press.

Secretaría de Gobernación. 2016. *NORMA Oficial Mexicana NOM-007-SSA2-2016, para la
atención de la mujer durante el embarazo, parto y puerperio, y de la persona recién nacida,*
July 4, 2016. www.dof.gob.mx/nota_detalle.php?codigo=5432289&fecha=07/04/2016.

Senado de la República: Coordinación de Comunicación Social. 2017. "La partería, en México,
es una práctica milenaria, reconocida en el mundo como una profesión." March 14, 2017.
comunicacion.senado.gob.mx/index.php/informacion/boletines/34997-la-parteria-en-
mexico-es-una-practica-milenaria-reconocida-en-el-mundo-como-una-profesion.html.

Sesia, Paola. 2017. "Maternal Death in Mexico." Edited by Oxford University Press. *Oxford Research Encyclopedia of Latin American History*, April 26, 2017. doi.org/10.1093/
acrefore/9780199366439.013.50.

Shakespeare, William. 2005. *Much Ado about Nothing*. New York: Penguin.

Simonds, Wendy, Barbara Katz Rothman, and Bari Meltzer Norman. 2006. *Laboring On:
Birth in Transition in the United States*. New York: Routledge.

Smith-Oka, Vania. 2012. "'They Don't Know Anything': How Medical Authority Constructs
Perceptions of Reproductive Risk among Low-Income Mothers in Mexico." In *Risk, Re-
production, and Narratives of Experience*, edited by L. Fordyce and A. Maraesa, 103–21.
Nashville, TN: Vanderbilt University Press.

———. 2013. "Managing Labor and Delivery among Impoverished Populations in Mexico:
Cervical Examinations as Bureaucratic Practice." *American Anthropologist* 115 (4):
595–607.

———. 2014. "Fallen Uterus: Social Suffering, Bodily Vigor, and Social Support among
Women in Rural Mexico." *Medical Anthropology Quarterly* 28 (1): 105–21. doi.org/10.1111/
maq.12064.

———. 2015 "Microaggressions and the Reproduction of Social Inequalities in Medical
Encounters in Mexico." *Social Science and Medicine* 143 (October): 9–16. doi.org/10.1016/J.
SOCSCIMED.2015.08.039.

Smith-Oka, Vania, and Megan K. Marshalla. 2019. "Crossing Bodily, Social, and Intimate
Boundaries: How Class, Ethnic, and Gender Differences Are Reproduced in Medical
Training in Mexico." *American Anthropologist* 121 (1): 113–25.

Smith-Oka, Vania, and Maryam Rokhideh. 2018. "Social Support and Social Suffering: Uterine Health and Isihuayo among Indigenous Women in Mexico." In *Maternal Death and
Pregnancy-Related Morbidity among Indigenous Women of Mexico and Central America*, edited by David A. Schwartz, 225–47. Cham, Switzerland: Springer International Publishing. doi.org/10.1007/978-3-319-71538-4_12.

Smith, Benjamin T. 2012. "Towards a Typology of Rural Responses to Healthcare in Mexico,
1920-1960." *Endeavour* 37 (1): 38–46.

Soto Laveaga, Gabriela. 2013. "Bringing the Revolution to Medical Schools: Social Service
and a Rural Health Emphasis in 1930s Mexico." *Mexican Studies/Estudios Mexicanos* 29
(2): 397–427. doi.org/10.1525/msem.2013.29.2.397.

Squires, Allison, and Adrián Juárez. 2012. "A Qualitative Study of the Work Environments of
Mexican Nurses." *International Journal of Nursing Studies* 49 (7): 793–802. doi.org/10.1016/j.
ijnurstu.2012.02.001.

Star, Susan Leigh. 1999. "The Ethnography of Infrastructure." *American Behavioral Scientist* 43 (3): 377–91. doi.org/10.1177/00027649921955326.

Summer, Anna, Dilys Walker, and Sylvia Guendelman. 2019. "A Review of the Forces Influencing Maternal Health Policies in Post-War Guatemala." *World Medical and Health Policy* 11 (1): 59–82. doi.org/10.1002/wmh3.292.

Thomasson, Melissa A., and Jaret Treber. 2008. "From Home to Hospital: The Evolution of Childbirth in the United States, 1928–1940." *Explorations in Economic History* 45 (1): 76–99. doi.org/10.1016/j.eeh.2007.07.001.

Tsing, Anna Lowenhaupt. 2005. *Friction: An Ethnography of Global Connection*. Princeton, NJ: Princeton University Press.

Tucker, Kathryn, Hector Ochoa, Rosario Garcia, Kirsty Sievwright, Amy Chambliss, and Margaret C. Baker. 2013. "The Acceptability and Feasibility of an Intercultural Birth Center in the Highlands of Chiapas, Mexico." *BMC Pregnancy and Childbirth* 13 (1): 94. doi.org/10.1186/1471-2393-13-94.

UN (United Nations). n.d. "Goal 3: Good Health and Well-Being | Sustainable Development Goals Fund." Accessed May 30, 2019. www.sdgfund.org/goal-3-good-health-and-well-being.

———. 1995. "Report of the International Conference on Population and Development." Cairo, September 5–13, 1994. New York: United Nations. www.un.org/en/development/desa/population/events/pdf/expert/27/SupportingDocuments/A_CONF.171_13_Rev.1.pdf

———. 2018. "Methodology." Statistics Division. unstats.un.org/unsd/methodology/m49.

UNFPA (United Nations Population Fund). 2006. "Investing in Midwives and Others with Midwifery Skills to Save the Lives of Mothers and Newborns and Improve Their Health: Policy and Programme Guidance for Countries Seeking to Scale up Midwifery Services, Especially at the Community Level." www.unfpa.org/sites/default/files/pub-pdf/midwives_eng.pdf.

Unger-Saldaña, K., A. Alvarez-Meneses, and D. Isla-Ortiz. 2018. "Symptomatic Presentation, Diagnostic Delays and Advanced Stage among Cervical Cancer Patients in Mexico." *Journal of Global Oncology* 4 (2): 221s. doi.org/10.1200/jgo.18.89600.

Van Hollen, Cecilia. 2003. *Birth on the Threshold: Childbirth and Modernity in South India*. Berkeley, CA: University of California Press.

———. 2011. "Breast or Bottle? HIV-Positive Women's Responses to Global Health Policy on Infant Feeding in India." *Medical Anthropology Quarterly* 25 (4): 499–518. doi.org/10.1111/j.1548-1387.2011.01182.x.

Vega, Rosalynn A. 2018. *No Alternative: Childbirth, Citizenship, and Indigenous Culture in Mexico*. Austin, TX: University of Texas Press.

Walzer Leavitt, Judith. 2016 [1986]. *Brought to Bed: Childbearing in America, 1750–1950*. New York: Oxford University Press.

Wendland, Claire. 2010. *A Heart for the Work: Journeys through an African Medical School*. Chicago, IL: University Of Chicago Press.

———. 2016. "Estimating Death: A Close Reading of Maternal Mortality Metrics in Malawi." In *Metrics: What Counts in Global Health*, edited by Vincanne Adams, 57–81. Durham, NC: Duke University Press.

Werner, David. 1980. *Donde no hay doctor: Una guía para los campesinos que viven lejos de los centros médicos*. Berkeley, CA: Herperian.

Wesp, Julie K. 2017. "Caring for Bodies or Simply Saving Souls: The Emergence of Institutional Care in Spanish Colonial America." In *New Developments in the Bioarchaeology of Care*, 253–76. Basel, Switzerland: Springer International Publishing. doi.org/10.1007/978-3-319-39901-0_13.

WHO (World Health Organization). n.d. "Maternal Mortality." Accessed September 30, 2019. www.who.int/news-room/fact-sheets/detail/maternal-mortality.

_____. 1997. "Care in Normal Birth: A Practical Guide. Report of a Technical Working Group." *Birth* 24 (2): 121–23. doi.org/10.1111/j.1523-536X.1997.00121.pp.x.

_____. 2004. "Making Pregnancy Safer: The Critical Role of the Skilled Attendant." A Joint Statement by WHO, ICM, and FIGO. Geneva: Department of Reproductive Health and Research, World Health Organization. apps.who.int/iris/bitstream/handle/10665/42955/9241591692.pdf.

_____. 2014. "Maternal Mortality Ratio (per 100,000 Live Births)." World Bank Open Data. data.worldbank.org.

_____. 2015a. "Health in 2015: From MDGs to SDGs." World Health Organization. www.who.int/gho/publications/mdgs-sdgs/en.

_____. 2015b. "WHO Statement on Caesarean Section Rates." World Health Organization. apps.who.int/iris/bitstream/handle/10665/161442/WHO_RHR_15.02_eng.pdf.

Williams, Sarah A. 2019. "Narratives of Responsibility: Maternal Mortality, Reproductive Governance, and Midwifery in Mexico." *Social Science and Medicine*, March 19, 2019. doi.org/10.1016/j.socscimed.2019.03.023.

Winskell, Kate, Peter J. Brown, Amy E. Patterson, Camilla Burkot, and Benjamin C. Mbakwem. 2013. "Making Sense of HIV in Southeastern Nigeria: Fictional Narratives, Cultural Meanings, and Methodologies in Medical Anthropology." *Medical Anthropology Quarterly* 27 (2): 193–214. doi.org/10.1111/maq.12023.

World Bank. 2019. "World Bank Country and Lending Groups." datahelpdesk.worldbank.org/knowledgebase/articles/906519-world-bank-country-and-lending-groups.

Zacher Dixon, Lydia. 2015. "Obstetrics in a Time of Violence: Mexican Midwives Critique Routine Hospital Practices." *Medical Anthropology Quarterly* 29 (4): 437–54. doi.org/10.1111/maq.12174.

Zhan, Mei. 2009. *Other-Worldly: Making Chinese Medicine through Transnational Frames.* Durham, NC: Duke University Press Books.

INDEX

Italicized page numbers refer to tables and illustrations